So You're "On Disability"

and you think you might want to get back into action

DANIEL
THOMAS MCANENY

TABLE OF CONTENTS

1. What It Means To You   1

2. Your Options - The Focus Is Yours To Choose   7

3. The Silver Lining   11

4. The Three-Stage Healing Framework   15

5. Getting Back To What?
   The Close Encounter Approach   21

6. Turning Obstacles To Advantages
   ..... In Your Head and In The World   23

7. Action ..... The Antidote To Isolation and
   The Key To The Opportunity Collision   43

8. Do You Want To Go Into Business?   57

9. Some People Who've Gotten Jobs,
   and Taught Me About ...   65

10. More People Who've Gotten Jobs,
    and Taught Me About ...   77

11. Still More People Who've Gotten Jobs,
    and Taught Me About ...   85

12. And Finally More People Who've Gotten Jobs,
    and Taught Me About ...   95

13. Some People Who Started Businesses
    ..... That Seemed To Fit   105

14. So Is There Anything In All Of This
    That Can Help You?   133

15. I'm Still Learning ..... Can You Help Me?   135
    Instructions for "Going Into Business" Forms

THANKS TO ...

...the hundreds of people who, after encountering a disability, touched and enriched my life, and taught me a lot in the process.

...the dozens of Vocational Rehabilitation and Customer Care Coordinators who have referred people to me over the years.

...the handful of special people in the profession who provided encouragement, feedback and support for this book.

...Jo Warner, Janis Truesdale and Bobbie Gibb, who got me started in this field.

...Meredith Young-Sowers and Stillpoint Publishing, Walpole NH, for the three-stage healing framework.

...Leo Buscaglia, for his unyielding commitment to love in its many forms. (Quote in Chapter 13 from *Born For Love,* by Leo F. Buscaglia, Ph.D., copyright 1992, by Leo F. Buscaglia, Inc., published by Slack, Inc.)

...Maureen, for tirelessly making copies, and Patty, for taking the flattering photo in the back of the first printing of this book, which photo is no longer available for reproduction.

FROM THE AUTHOR TO THE READER

One day about a year ago it occurred to me that there are certain things I've repeated to clients over the years that seemed to help them. My clients are people who are receiving benefits under long term disability income policies, and want to "get back into action," either by finding a job or getting into a business.

The insurance companies pay me to assist them, in what is a totally voluntary effort on the part of the person receiving benefits. My "customers" in the insurance companies often have a title such as "Vocational Rehabilitation Coordinator," and many of them have completed several post-graduate courses of study, and earned various professional designations, which equip them to assist people in a number of ways.

Working with them over the past nine years has been a pure joy. Their motivation is to help people on disability who want to return to a more productive and meaningful daily work effort. To do that they skillfully orchestrate the talents of many different types of organizations, of which mine is only one. And while it is true that insurors can and usually do benefit financially when a person returns to work or builds a successful business, my customers don't let that get in the way of acting in my clients' best interests at all times.

As you know, there are many departments and functions within any insurance company. You may have already dealt with some people whose job it is to verify the validity of your claim. In the process they may have challenged some of your statements or requested additional medical examinations, and your relationships with them may or may not have been pleasant.

When and if you deal with a Vocational Rehabilitation Coordinator, however, you are dealing with someone whose job it is to assist you, if you are motivated and capable of some type of work activity. You can expect that any interaction with them will be positive and helpful. So if you think you might want to get back into action, but you're not sure, you'd be well advised to check whether your policy provides for Vocational Rehabilitation services, and if so, ask to speak with someone in that department.

As I mentioned, many of my clients have found some of the things I've said to be comforting or encouraging, but the number of people I work with is just a tiny fraction of the number contacted by my customers. So why not, I reasoned, put some of these thoughts down in writing, and add some stories to serve as examples, so that a far greater number of people on disability could be exposed to them?

The result is this book, and its sole intent is to provide some thoughts, some perspectives, and some stories, that a person on long term disability might find helpful in some way. I'm well aware, however, that what one person finds helpful, another may find offensive. So if any of the perspectives presented here offend you, or if the stories of others' successes are for you disheartening rather than uplifting, please stop reading, put the book down, and accept my apologies for the intrusion on your day.

If on the other hand you can find just one thought or story that provides reassurance or encouragement, then I thank you for being there to graciously receive it, and for fulfilling the purpose of the book.

This Book Is Dedicated To Mae McAneny,
Who Was Supposed To Die At 6,
But Who Hung Around An Additional 92 Years
And Managed To Do A Lot Of Good Things
Before Leaving Us.

1.
WHAT IT MEANS TO YOU

Bill had been a high-powered financial wholesaler for many years before his heart attack, selling financial products to other financial professionals. When I met him in Boston he had been out for only a year, and looked in perfect health. He was still young, in his late thirties, and the attack had scared him. So he had stopped drinking, dieted religiously, and exercised regularly. It was now time for him to take those first steps toward getting back to work.

But mentally he wasn't ready yet. "Dan, nobody knows what it means, what it does to your life. I've kept in close touch with my friends, lunch almost every week, and I've tried to explain it to them, but there are no words. The boredom and frustration are bad enough. But you also begin to feel strange, as though what you used to do somehow isn't real anymore. The world seems different, and you're not sure you fit in it, the way you did before the disability."

Fred, a brilliant manufacturing engineer, had been out for five years. He had relocated from California to Tennessee to lower his living costs. He had made key contributions in the design and manufacture of products as diverse as tin cans and helicopters. After five years, he was still eager to get back to work, and not just because he needed to earn more money.

"The financial problems are big," I remember him telling me, "and I'm still dealing with back and leg pains. But what really gets me is that I don't have those interesting engineering projects anymore. It was a lot of fun figuring out creative answers to tough design problems, and I guess I was spoiled. It's not easy to fill your day when you're used to doing what you love, then you can't do it anymore."

The story is the same even when the job isn't ideal. Consider the words of Orlando, who had held a job in electronics assembly before his back problems got worse. "I never thought I had an especially good job, but now I realize how much I miss seeing those people every day, joking around, even working extra fast when we had to. That job looks pretty good to me now." Phil, who had been a janitor before eye problems developed, felt the same way. "Looking back, Dan, I see I enjoyed it in ways I didn't even know, but you could never have convinced me of that back then."

No one but you can know what your disability means to you. Not even another person with a long term disability. Life with a disability is just as individualized and isolated as the healthy life you had before it happened. How can anyone else truly understand your particular blend of frustrations, anxieties, determination, hopes, fears, and all the subtle shades of emotions, or lack of them, in between?

If you're on long term disability, it's likely that at one time, maybe not that long ago, you were working ..... either for an employer, in your profession, or in your own business. You were healthy enough to do your job, and to some degree you identified with that job. You may have had the normal degree of discontent, or you may have loved it. Regardless, it gave you a place to go, useful and productive things to do, and at some level, a comfortable feeling that, however important or unimportant you were in the overall scheme of things, you fit in.

You were a functioning part of the world of commerce, a cog in the wheel of the great machine that makes the world hum. You were doing your part, however exalted or humble, in producing the goods and services that we all sell to one another to keep ourselves fed and clothed and housed.

And you felt pretty good about it. Or if not, at least it provided activity and filled your days with challenges, or problems to solve, or interactions with others. You had talents and you were using them, perhaps to create something, sell something, operate something, analyze something, make something happen, help others make something happen, or maybe stop something from happening. It gave you a place to be and things to do that the rest of the world respected as honest labor, whatever its status.

But suddenly, one day, everyone else is going to work ..... and you're not. Maybe it was because of an accident. Maybe it was an illness or physical problem that gradually, or suddenly, got worse. Maybe it was a stroke. Or maybe it was an operation that didn't go right. Whatever, it left you unable to perform as you always had ..... and as you had always taken for granted.

That first day when you couldn't go to work like everyone else, the world shifted slightly on you. You perceived it from an angle you'd never quite experienced before. Things weren't the same, and it was uncomfortable somehow. On the second day, they shifted a little bit more.

Gradually, with each passing day, you begin to inhabit a different psychological space. You're not addressing the world the way you did for so long. Questions may arise. Who am I, if I'm no longer the person who does such-and-such each day? Am I still lovable if I'm no longer out there achieving and producing? Just what is the significance of my life?

Concerns may start to surface. Will I ever be productive

again? Can I be happy doing something different from what I've always done? How far am I falling behind? How will my family get by? Will I become a burden, or worse yet, a bore?

Depending on your answers to those kinds of questions, you may gradually regain peace of mind and a healthy level of self-esteem ..... or things may go the other way.

By the time six months pass, you might be in any number of emotional places. For some, they fully expect to be "back in the swing of things" in some specified time period, and they keep themselves occupied by staying up-to-date in their chosen field. No problem there.

For others, however, it might be a little more complicated. Maybe they realize they can't go back to doing what they used to do any time soon ..... or ever. Maybe they realize their employer doesn't want them back or can't make room for them. Or they can't go back to running their business as they had. Maybe they develop a real sense of isolation, not knowing anyone else in their set of particularly difficult circumstances.

Financial problems often develop, even with the cushion of benefit payments from their disability income policy. Marital and other relationships are tested, and sometimes it turns out to be a destructive test. Friends may not know how to respond properly, and slowly slip away. Wives or husbands may not be able to handle the pressure, and there can be a lot of pressure. Problems here.

If there's pain -- really bad pain -- it can mean very big problems. Your whole world becomes focused on how to live with that pain. The energy and concentration it takes can be all-consuming, leaving little else of life to be experienced, none of it savored. And if you need to take drugs to help you cope with it, they can rob you of that clear conscious focus on life you'd always assumed would be yours, rob you of your energy, your stamina, your zest for life.

So depending upon your circumstances, your reactions, and your individual makeup, a disability can mean just a temporary setback, or it can bring your whole world crashing down around you, tearing apart the whole fabric of your existence, erasing all the familiar reference points by which you judged your daily experience, and distorting all the standards and many of the values you relied on to assign meaning to your life.

And only you can truly know what it means to you. So if someone tells you they understand your situation because they've worked with hundreds of others in similar circumstances, or because they've "gone through it themselves" at some point, you might choose to forgive their presumptuousness, and appreciate that they mean well.

But you know they don't *really* know. They don't *really* understand. You know what though? In terms of whether their understanding helps you get out of this place you're in, to some other place you'd rather be, you might ask the question, what difference does it make? You have your options regardless.

2.

YOUR OPTIONS -- THE FOCUS IS YOURS
TO CHOOSE

Over the years I've done a lot of different things for a lot of people on disability, and it can be a humbling experience. Makes you realize firsthand the meaning of one of the many lines Clint Eastwood made famous, "A man's got to know his limitations."

In my business, if you're not careful, you can fall into the trap of thinking that somehow, by doing the things you do, you are playing a big role in improving someone else's life. Experience has long since taught me, I'm at most a bit player in the drama of someone else's earthly existence.

I do what I do. Person A will take it and use it as one part of their overall efforts to make something great happen. Person B will ignore it and nothing happens. Person C will ignore it and make something great happen anyway. Person D might use some of it, or all of it, and something mediocre happens.

It's up to them, to you, to each of us, to be masters of our own fate. Never has this been made clearer to me than in working with people on disability. Thrown up against some of the toughest challenges any of us have to face in these closing years of the 20th century in the U.S.A., these people clearly choose from an infinitely wide range of reactions and focuses available to them, to plot the particular course that they alone will determine.

The nature and severity of the disability matters little. Those determined to get back to a productive life in the world of industry and commerce will do so, using whatever I and others might provide along the way to assist them. Those determined to devote their lives to volunteer and charitable work will do so. Those determined to achieve peace of mind without working, while enduring pain most of us can't imagine, will do so.

And those who are intent on remaining bitter, choosing to focus on the negative aspects of their experience, will find that those negative aspects occupy more and more of their daily existence. It's not my place to judge them, or try to place some moral value on anyone's choice of focus. They're taking on challenges that most of us would hope never to have to face.

But after a while, when you've gotten close to hundreds of people who have taken on these tough challenges, it becomes apparent that, even within the framework of the much narrower options available to them after a disability, it is their personal will and personal choice of focus that takes them along a specific path for which they alone are responsible.

And however grand or menial that path may seem to the outside observer, it is they alone who will determine how much satisfaction, peace of mind, joy, or frustration they will glean from it. They set their own parameters for what they will do, and what it will mean to them. At some point they come to realize that the only person who will be hurt or rewarded by their choice of focus is they themselves.

One of the most striking examples of someone who simply put his past behind him and determined to find satisfaction in a new career was a former tugboat captain, Tom A. Tom had relocated back to West Virginia after an accident, which resulted in back injuries severe enough so that he could no longer do what he loved best.

Now when you love being a tugboat captain, it's hard to find satisfaction in most other ways of living. But this fellow was determined, and he had a way of looking on the bright side. A lot of people in his situation might figure they were too specialized for anyone else to hire them, but not Tom.

He agreed with me that he had in effect been managing a demanding service business that required quick thinking, dealing with all sorts of people under sometimes difficult circumstances, training others to perform at the top of their ability, and maintaining "facilities" and equipment in top condition.

As he saw it, that's precisely what is required for profitably managing many types of businesses. When he succeeded in winning an offer to manage a newly opened "super drug store" in a town 20 miles away, he jumped at it. He was still quite happy six months later. He enjoyed developing people, building their confidence, and this job gave him that opportunity, along with other challenges.

Tom and I worked by phone, so we never met personally. He told me he was small in stature, but that the fellow who hired him had told him, "You know, you're a small fellow, but you have a big spirit. The way you project energy and confidence, before I met you, I figured you were twice the size. How could I not hire you?"

The people I get to work with, like Tom, are for the most part those who have already decided that they want to make real in their lives a sense of joy, achievement, and fulfillment. They want to get back in the fracas, doing the best they can at whatever it is they are now capable of doing, willing to take whatever ups and downs come with the territory. And they've taught me a lot. Like the Silver Lining, for example.

3.
THE SILVER LINING

It was difficult deciding when to address this, because it's a sensitive subject, and it may offend some people. But it's not my conclusion after all, so I suppose I shouldn't be hesitant, and decided to put it up front here. The first few times I heard people tell me this, I thought it was interesting. By the 100th time, I figured there was some lesson to be learned here, perhaps an intimation of some great truth, that warranted putting it in writing. So here it is.

"Dan, I would never knowingly wish this disability on myself, but in retrospect I have to say there have been some good things that came from it. Some important things. There has been a silver lining to this cloud."

In so many words, that's the common theme. From there, they branch off into different particulars. Some say they've become more patient, some more understanding of people with certain traits. Some feel they've got their values and priorities in line for the first time. Some have learned to cherish and enjoy seemingly small pleasures in life that previously they weren't aware of. Some discovered an emotional side to themselves, or a depth of understanding, that they didn't know existed.

Where it gets really interesting, and where some people might get offended, is when they comment on the meaning of this event within the overall perspective of their lives. What it comes down to is this. They've come to the conclusion, or they already knew, they say, that life is to be lived as a learning and growing experiece, and so the disability was an opportunity to do some learning and growing.

Further, they generally believe that at some level, they accepted this challenge so it could teach them something or bring them a more mature outlook on life. Depending on their religious persuasion or lack of it, they might refer to their subconscious, or Divine Providence, or the powers that be, or God, or the Universe, or the Good Lord, or their Oversoul, but the point remains the same.

They have accepted the challenge, the reasoning goes, and it is up to them to make the most of it. Now I hope never to have to address that issue firsthand as they have ..... probably wouldn't have the courage. I'm quick to tell them that I'm happy to learn my lessons in this life as an observer, learning from others' suffering as they relate their hard-won wisdom to me. It's usually good for a chuckle when I repeat my philosophy on that, a line borrowed from a favorite author, "Suffering is only good for the soul if it teaches you how to stop suffering."

The client who probably believed most fervently in the Silver Lining, Dave B, had been a partner in a public relations firm in the southeast, who had suffered a stroke at the height of a successful career. I remember the phone call when he joked about it being a "stroke of good luck."

As he put it, the stroke had forced some changes in relationships which were good for all concerned, and he had a new appreciation for the "spiritual" side of life that he hadn't even been aware of previously. He got an enjoyment out of helping other people now, that was unmatched by the joy of his business achievements.

When last I spoke with him, some of the effects of the stroke were still evident, but it wasn't slowing him down. He was touring his favorite parts of the country, checking out businesses to purchase that would suit his new priorities.

There are some interesting implications to the Silver Lining perspective that people like Dave adopt. It certainly puts them in control of the situation. And if the lesson has been learned, as one of them told me, they no longer have any need for the disease. They can let go of it, and eventually its symptoms may leave also. I happen to admire that belief structure, but whether you do or not, you've got to admit, it certainly serves the believer quite well in terms of inspiring hope, and maintaining a positive outlook.

Which brings you to the obvious question. What's the alternative? I could be missing something here, but it seems the alternative would be to see yourself as a victim, laid low by chance, with no apparent rhyme or reason for the illness or accident striking you instead of the next guy. That could be very tough to live with. It's easy to understand how someone could become quite bitter with that belief system. "Why me?" And never a really good answer, day after day, year after year.

Other than the fact that the Silver Lining perspective seems to work well for a lot of people, I make no value judgments. It's presented here as an interesting perspective. I remember though, years ago, when a young medical doctor with intense headaches expressed her absolute rage at "some new age people" who tried to tell her that she was "creating her own reality." "As if I don't feel horrible enough about this already," she said, "the thought that I'm doing it to myself would make me feel guilty and drive me insane."

She was the one suffering the intense daily pain of headaches, not her "new age" acquaintances, and no comforting thoughts for her came readily to mind. As much as I like the perspective of the Silver Lining, I don't think she would have appreciated it. It's easy to understand her perspective.

Who knows, you or I might have the same reaction, having to put up with that kind of pain. Few people are tested that drastically. Fortunately, most of the people I deal with, unlike that doctor, are well enough to function in some kind of work, and are motivated to do so. For them, there is another framework that often proves helpful. The name that's evolved for it is *The Three-Stage Healing Framework*.

4.
THE THREE-STAGE HEALING FRAMEWORK

Even for people who are very motivated to return to meaningful productive activity, one very significant obstacle is the feeling that the time since the onset of their disability has been wasted time, time that has been lost and can never be regained.

Fortunately this just isn't so. It may appear to be so, if you look only at surface events. But there is a healing perspective I read about years ago (I have almost no original ideas) in a book by a woman named Meredith Lady Young, that I found applied to many of my clients. When I share it with new clients, it often makes a lot of sense to them, and helps them shift their focus ... away from the frustration of "wasted time" ... to the anticipation of exploring new opportunities.

This perspective looks at the entire time from their disability to their getting back into a productive and fulfilling life, as a healing process with three stages. The first stage is not one where the person immediately goes out and starts knocking on the world's door, expecting to get into action right away.

Stage 1 ..... Making The Internal Adjustments

Instead, it is essentially an internal process. There is a

lot of internal work done here, as the person gradually gets adjusted to a dramatically new set of circumstances, and tries to regain some equilibrium and get their balance, so to speak, as new roles, new limitations, and new ground rules for daily existence are thrust upon them.

This is hard work, and the person who comes through it without being defeated, with a determination to get back to meaningful and rewarding daily activity, can be very proud indeed of this achievement. It's really the phase where the challenge is the greatest, where the most work is done, and the most progress made. Those who come through it intact are truly survivors. The fact that the work is primarily internal, rather than external, does not detract from its significance.

As soon as people realize this has been true in their own case, they understand that they knew it all along. It just took someone else's saying it for them, to acknowledge openly what they already knew internally. When they do acknowledge it, they are often immediately freed from the energy-consuming focus on having "wasted all this time." They understand instead that they have successfully met one of life's greatest challenges.

They don't even have to think about it. It's as though a little explosion goes off. They are filled with excitement, anticipation, and a new surge of energy. As one person put it, he was suddenly "galvanized into action." A great burden is lifted from their shoulders, as they realize that all along, getting rid of the burden was as easy as simply putting it down.

The realization dawns, "Hey, I haven't been wasting time, I've been doing great things. Let's get on with it !! "

For some people this first stage can take only a matter of weeks. For others, it's a matter of months. And for quite a few, it can take years. There are no rules about the "right amount of time," but people know when it's time. Their frustration and anxiety start to grow. They start to think more and more about how they're going to "get back into action," and what they might find to do that will be appealing and rewarding.

Even when they know that getting back into action may result in their eventually having a lot less security than they have on disability payments, their need to live what they consider a meaningful life outweighs those concerns. They're willing to take the risk. Fortunately, most disability policies have provisions that can help minimize that risk, and make it a very calculated one indeed.

Stage 2 ..... Finding Something To Get Excited About

It is usually when people are coming to the end of this first stage that I get involved. They are ready for the second stage, which is *finding something to get excited about.* When people find a direction they can get excited about, it unleashes their positive energies. They can then focus all their actions on attaining a goal that they feel is worthwhile. They begin to see their actions as no longer fractionated, without a consistent purpose. Instead, they start to feel a steady surge of well-directed energy, like a laser beam going after a specific target with a tremendous amount of concentrated power.

For people who've been on disability for a while, it can be a particularly tough challenge to find something to get excited about, and we'll touch shortly on one approach that's helpful for moving them through this stage.

Stage 3 ..... Opening Up To The World In A Mutual Give-and-Take

The third stage in this healing framework is *opening up to the world in a mutual give-and-take effort* aimed at reaching the goal. The person continues to *give* to others whenever possible, but also learns to *receive* graciously from others, letting them help in the effort and thereby enjoy the good feelings that come from being a giver. This mutual interchange of positive energies in the give-and-take is what completes the healing, both on the spiritual and physical levels.

So it is not reaching the goal itself, but the process of getting there, that completes the healing. For what it's worth, about 90% of my clients turn out to be people who have always been givers, and have no problems with that role, but have never learned to be gracious receivers.

When they begin to realize how much others gain when they are allowed to be givers, they understand that they've been cutting off half the energy flow that is natural among humans, and they gain greater appreciation for the natural healing effects of a smooth, two-way flow of that energy.

And the timing is quite fortunate for learning that lesson. Whenever you are attempting to get a job or start a business that is different from what you've done before, you can use all the help that might come your way. This third stage usually unfolds according to an action plan that we figure out up front, so that the person gets the feeling of a systematic buildup of momentum, with no wasted motion.

The client who reacted most dramatically to experiencing the two-way flow of energy in the third stage was Paul T, who lived in the Boston area. Paul had an excellent record of achievement in materials management and inventory control, when he suffered a stroke that left him with almost no mobility, and many other functions severely impaired.

In addition to his full-time job, Paul had also been a part-time entertainer in the evenings and on weekends, performing an outstanding one-man show as a singer and musician who impersonated Neil Diamond and Elvis. He was so good that he raised $30,000 for a charity in just four shows on consecutive evenings.

Among his many fine qualities, Paul was very determined, and he surprised a lot of people by walking out of the hospital when a number of medical professionals had told him he'd probably spend the rest of his life maneuvering from a wheelchair. When I met him, he was dragging a leg, and one arm drooped, but he was walking.

We agreed to start a job search for a materials management position. I emphasized how important it would be for him to open himself up and let others help him, knowing it would be difficult for him. He had always been strong and independent, the classic giver who still had to learn how to be a gracious receiver.

He responded beautifully, and kept himself open to receiving assistance from many sources. He enjoyed the process, especially as he saw how pleased others were when they could help him. The job search was turning up opportunities, and while he hadn't gotten an offer yet, he was building momentum. So much so, that he confided to me he wanted to start singing again to audiences, and he showed me some pages he had written about his experiences.

I was impressed with his writing and his singing, and encouraged him to continue with both. His story had the potential to inspire a lot of people. The point was also made that his singing could entertain others and give him a lot of joy at the same time. That was all the encouragement Paul needed.

Within a few months he was putting on a one-hour show for stroke and accident victims in area hospitals and other recovery facilities. A major TV station in Boston found out about him and featured him on their "Hero" series. The resulting publicity led to his singing the national anthem before 30,000 people at Fenway Park in Boston. He completed his inspirational book, and a local civic group is sponsoring the printing of it, for distribution to anyone in the area who has suffered a stroke or has limited mobility as a result of an accident.

Financially, from an insuror's point of view, Paul's case is not ideal. He may or may not find another job in materials handling. He'd like to. He came in #2 for a very good job about the time he appeared at Fenway. But from the perspective of helping someone regain a positive spirit, the insuror can count this as an unqualified success. Paul is the first to tell you, the mutual exchange of energy in giving and receiving has lifted his life to a new level. The feelings he gets from giving his performances, and from letting others help him as he does, are so rejuvenating to his spirit that he knows this is one of the things he was meant to do in life.

5.

GETTING BACK TO ..... WHAT?
The *Close Encounter* Approach

In discussing the three-stage healing process, the point was made that, for people on disability, the second stage, finding something to get excited about, can be difficult.

In fact, a lot of people beat themselves up because they aren't able to generate a lot of enthusiasm for some new goal. They shouldn't. If they think about it, they would start to understand that it's unrealistic to expect themselves to get excited about something they've never done before. And while significant strides are being made in workplace adaptations and assistive devices that help people return to previous occupations, many of those on long term disability need to find something to do that they haven't done before.

For those people, anything they contemplate is bound to be something they've never really gotten close to. Do you know anyone who can get truly excited about something they've never gotten close to? The answer here is to release yourself from the unrealistic expectation that you can get excited about something at a distance.

Instead, we identify things a person thinks they *might get excited about if they got close to them.* Then we provide them whatever they need to get closer to those goals, to find out for themselves firsthand whether they still want them when they are up close. We call it *Close Encounter With Stated Goals.* Very important here is the perspective, which says that if they get close to a goal and find they don't like it, *that's real progress!!*

Why? Because we've eliminated a "phantom goal," which allows them to focus their energies more clearly on another goal. In the meantime, they are developing a better understanding of what they really want, based on real-life experiences, not just on guesses made at a distance.

Once people understand that it's okay to go after something, find they don't like it, drop it, and pursue something else, they lose a lot of their anxiety and are able to make real progress. It isn't even something they have to think about. Their *feelings* tell them soon enough whether a particular option is going to be right for them. The whole process flows more smoothly and naturally.

This *Close Encounter* approach enables people to seek out and discard a number of options, if necessary, without feeling guilty or pressured about it. And the funny thing is, with all that freedom to pursue endlessly, few people go through more than two or three options without finding the one that they *know* is right for them. Sometimes it takes a while, and sometimes they complete the process quickly.

You may be concerned that if you try this, you may have endless *close encounters.* My advice? Press on anyway. If that were to happen, it may mean you have some fears you haven't yet recognized, and at some point you'll need to face them. Maybe you aren't as motivated as you think, which is helpful to discover. Or maybe you just haven't yet found the option that's right for you. The only way to find the answer is to keep on moving ahead.

6.

TURNING OBSTACLES TO ADVANTAGES

·····

In Your Head And In the World

An essential part of feeling good about any option, is believing that you are qualified for it, that you can make contributions in that role, and that if anyone has concerns or objections about you, you can deal effectively with those concerns. If you can't do that, it's difficult to develop much self-confidence, and without a lot of confidence, it's difficult to reach a goal.

So one of the things we need to deal with up front is the question of problems, concerns, and limitations -- real or perceived. At the outset of my work with clients, they are usually asked to complete my information-surfacing forms. These forms ask people to tell about the good things they've done *and how they've done them.* (The forms help them figure this out if they're not sure.)

That information helps me understand how they address the world, and which strengths they normally rely on to get things done. That in turn helps us figure out which options might hold the most appeal for them, and provides lots of raw material for creating resumes, brochures, credentials summaries, or whatever else they might need to help them get closer to a goal.

But the forms also ask them to tell about their concerns,

and any objections they think they might encounter. This is especially important where people are seeking jobs instead of starting a business. Anyone with a long term disability is invariably going to have a few basic concerns about objections from employers. These concerns will keep them from becoming truly confident until they figure out how to handle them. So let's take a look at the most common ones.

"What have you been doing lately?"

By far the potential question that conjures up the most negative images ... and causes the most dread ... is, "What have you been doing for the past ..... (two years), (ten months), (six years) ....?" Your lack of recent employment may or may not be evident on your resume, but you can expect the question to arise naturally in the course of conversation sooner or later.

Most people imagine themselves talking about the disability, followed perhaps by an awkward silence for a few moments, followed by more questions.

They see themselves losing hope as the focus shifts from what they might do for the company, to how their disability might affect their performance. Even if the interviewer's concerns aren't actually spoken, the person coming back from a disability imagines them, and becomes defensive. In their own mind, they've already lost it, which means in fact they have.

The root of the solution here is not to try to neutralize, defend, or explain. You can only lose that way. To use an anlogy with football, it is as though you were playing the entire game between the 50-yard line and the end zone you are defending. At best you might keep the other team from scoring, but you can never score any points, never win.

If you are to have any chance of coming out a winner in this discussion, you absolutely must turn this to an advantage. That's right, an advantage. If you can't come to sincerely believe that, don't even try, because it won't work. So the place to start with this objection is in your own head, to see what you believe.

How can it be perceived as an advantage? How can you start talking about it by claiming it's the single strongest reason they should hire you? Let's start with the observable facts.

If you're actually out there looking for a job, it means you've come through your disability a victor, doesn't it? Where others might have given up and gotten discouraged, you persevered. You recovered to the point where you can function again, and had the guts to go out into the world, risk rejection and perhaps some financial security, and start knocking on doors.

In the process you may have reached deep inside and developed personal strengths you never knew you had. And certainly you've overcome a huge challenge. By virtue of what you've gone through, you know you can achieve anything if you put your mind to it, regardless of the odds. So it's likely you're more determined than the average person, with a can-do attitude born of firsthand experience. True?

A wonderful quality to have in an employee. True?

But that's not all. You've had time to think about all the things you might want to do. And you don't have to go out and find a job if you prefer not to. But of your own choosing you are out there looking for a job. And of all the things you might want to do, the one job you are seeking is the one you're interviewing for.

Talk about an employee coming to a position with a clear idea of what he or she wants!

No second guessing here. No exits two weeks later because you decided you wanted something else. We're talking about commitment, one of the most important traits any employer looks for.

There's more. You've been out for a while. The inactivity frustrated you beyond words. Yes, you achieved a victory over an unfortunate event, but that victory won't be complete until you're back into a productive, satisfying job, where you know you'll be contributing.

Simply for having gone through your disability experience, you value a job more highly than the next person. Getting back into action and turning in outstanding performance means a lot more to you than it possibly could to anyone else they might consider.

That means you'll be more highly motivated than anyone else.

More highly motivated? More enthused about turning in a great performance? Is that the single most important factor for many employers when making a hiring decision? Yes it is. And you've got it.

Unusual personal strengths, determination, commitment, motivation. Pretty strong qualifiers, I'd say. And true for most people on disability that I've worked with. If you agree that these facts are true in your case, you would do well to internalize them. Come to believe them as strongly as you believe anything. Because if you are going to have others out there in the world of employment agree with you, you're going to have to believe it yourself first.

One exercise that might help you is to take a pocket recorder, and rehearse how you'd answer the question, "What have you been doing for the last _____ years?" Start with a phrase like, "I'm glad you asked. What I've been doing the last _____ years, and what I've achieved, probably constitutes the single strongest reason you should hire me. Let me explain."

Follow up with your personalized version of the general truths you agreed to in the previous paragraphs, if you agreed with them, and conclude with the feedback question, "Do you see now why I say that what I've done during the past _____ years is the single strongest reason you should hire me?"

Somehow, working out loud with the words reinforces your own belief in these truths, and strengthens your resolve to get out there and convice some employer that you really are the best person to hire. And even if you don't convince everyone, it feels really good to play in the other fellow's half of the field. Do it enough and the law of numbers starts to work for you. If 10 people hear this, it's likely that at least one will agree, and maybe even be very impressed. You only need one.

In case you're wondering, yes, a lot of my clients have used this over the years, including a number who at first didn't really believe it. It has not worked every time. It has worked *some* of the time for *every* person who tried it more than once. Sounds like that famous line about "fooling some of the people," doesn't it? Except you're not fooling.

"You haven't done this type of work before."

Let's look at another common concern. When you're on disability, almost by definition, you aren't able to function in the job you held previously. So whatever you're going after, it stands to reason you haven't done it before. A potential legitimate concern, therefore, might be phrased this way by an employer .....

"Judy, you've got an admirable record of achievement, and some of your experience fits, but we do have one strong reservation, and it's the fact that you haven't done this particular type of work before."

Now believe it or not, your answer is not the most important thing here. It is not the focus of this book to go deeply into the interview process, but essentially interviewing is a matter of establishing rapport, then finding out what the employer needs and letting them know you have it. Concerns like this one usually come up after you've done all that.

Which means you've probably built up a certain positive momentum if you've gotten that far. You obviously don't want to lose that. But the natural reaction here is either to agree, which doesn't help, or to get defensive, and argue the point that your experience does fit. Problem is, even if you win the "argument," you lose the rapport, and very likely the job offer as well.

The solution? Recognize first that if someone raises an objection, it's a positive sign. Employers don't waste time raising objections about people they're not interested in. And if someone is straightforward enough to lay their objection right out for you, that's something to be appreciated, because now you can deal with it.

Next you need to understand that hiring is largely a *psychological* process, where *emotions* get involved. If it were strictly logical, computers could do it. So what happens *psychologically and emotionally* here is far more important than what happens *logically and intellectually.*

If you've built up rapport, you don't want to lose it by arguing. So your answer to the objection should not be given right away. That's too much like a rebuttal. Instead, try following a simple 4-step process where the first three steps are psychologically based, and you don't get to your answer until step #4.

In Step #1 you simply acknowledge that this is indeed something you should be talking about. Why? Well, the first thing that happens when someone raises an objection, however politely, is that the tension rises. This brings the tension back down.

"I can appreciate your concern. Thanks for being straightforward in telling me directly. If I were in your position, I think I might raise the same issue."

Step #2 *redirects* the conversation away from the stated concern, toward the corresponding positives, which are the positive things the employer is looking for, that caused them to raise their concern in the first place.

"I understand when you raise that concern, you want to be sure the person you put in this job is able to come in and start contributing right away, isn't that it?"

Notice that this comment also turns the conversation away from you, and toward some hypothetical ideal person, making the discussion less personal, more objective, and therefore more comfortable. It ends with a question so you don't have to do all the talking, and you give the other person a chance to say something positive. That person may also feel good about your ability to understand so thoroughly the basis for raising the concern. The reply is likely to be:

"That's right. That's precisely why I brought it up. You obviously understand."

Step #3 is to ask whether, if you could show you have those positive qualities, it might ease their concern somewhat.

"If I could share a few thoughts with you that would show I have those qualities and could probably contribute quickly, might that help ease your concern a little?"

The question is phrased in a way that makes it very easy for someone to say "yes." It also gives the other person a chance to say something, so you have a bit of a back-and-forth conversation that takes you still further from that initial tension that arose when the concern was raised.

Now you're ready for Step #4, your answer, and in truth it doesn't matter that much how effective the actual answer is. The key thing is that the other person realizes, at some level, that you handled the objection pretty well, and didn't get flustered or argumentative. You win regardless.

Your answer can follow a number of strategies that have worked for people over the years. Often it's very effective to have a story ready about a similar situation in the past, where you faced challenges you hadn't dealt with previously, but surprised a lot of people by making contributions almost immediately. After the story, ask a feedback question, to bring closure to the discussion, hopefully again on a positive note.

"Does that help show I might have the kind of flexibility, and quickness to contribute, that you are looking for here?"

Any Job Can Be Broken Into Component Parts

If you don't have a story, another effective type of answer is to show that, while you've never had that particular job, at one time or another you have had experience in all the component parts of the job. Any job can be broken down into its component parts, and so, for example, you may not have managed a distribution department before, but you might be able to show you've had direct experience in shipping, receiving, setting up systems to control shipments and order processing, and in managing a different department.

The point could be made that, because, at one time or another, you did a good job in each of the component functions, you're confident that you could perform well in this job. Again, close with the feedback question.

"I'm a member of that group"

Still another way to answer in Step #4 is to use the *"I'm a member of that group" approach.* We can define ourselves narrowly or broadly. When you have the specific experience someone is looking for, it pays to define yourself narrowly as a member of a small group having that particular background, because you are that specialist who fits all the criteria. But for the objection we're dealing with here, it pays to define yourself as a member of a bigger group.

So imagine a series of concentric cicles. In the center is a small circle which defines you very narrowly, for example, as *Quality Control Manager for Electromechanical Components in Simulation Systems.*

By virtue of being that, you are part of a larger group, which includes *All QC Managers for Electromechanical Components,* regardless of what systems they may be part of. When you think about it, you could also be defined as being part of .....

All QC Managers for Components, electromechanical, or whether they are electronic, mechanical

All QC Managers, whether for components, systems, or subsystems

All Managers of Manufacturing Functions, whether QC, Design, Production, etc.

All Managers of any Functions in a Manufacturing Company

All Managers in any Type of Company

All People Who Have Held Responsible Positions in Business
All People Who Have Held Responsible Positions in Any Organization

And so on, until you get to the largest group, which is *human being.* It's important to remember that you can draw parallels between your experience and what an employer is looking for, *at any of these levels.*

You might make the point that they are looking for a *Manager of a Manufacturing Function,* (in this case the 5th level), that you are a member of that group and do indeed have that experience, and that you learn quickly. That means you'd be up to speed in a very short time by learning in the first few weeks whatever you need to learn, in order to do an outstanding job. Again, the feedback question comes at the end.

So you've got lots of options for your answer in Step #4, but a good answer will require some preparation. You may find the information-surfacing forms helpful in preparing stories about good things you've done in the past, in breaking your jobs into component parts, and figuring out levels of specialism. If you'd like to work with those forms, your insuror might be able to provide them. If not, instructions for ordering them can be found in the back of this book.

"You're not up-to-date on recent developments."

Now let's turn to a third common concern for anyone on long term disability. It can be phrased in a number of ways, but in so many words it comes down to:

"You've been out for _____ years. The industry has made a lot of advances in that time. Don't you think you'd be a little rusty?"

The fact is, you may be. So the time to address this concern is before you ever get to an interview. One way to quickly update yourself on industry trends is to read a dozen or so back issues of the leading trade magazines. They might be available at a large library with a business reference section. If not, consult the *SRDS Business Publications Rates & Data,* a reference source available in most libraries that gives you contact information on all trade magazines. Call the magazines directly for advice on how to get access to back issues.

If you don't have time for that, for a quickie update check out the *Predicasts F&S Index,* either on computer or in print at most good reference libraries. It's arranged by SIC Code, and gives you the headlines of all important articles that have been printed in the past year in trade magazines that correspond to a particular SIC Code.

The SIC Code is the government's Standard Industrial Classification Code. It is a numerical code system, and every type of business will have an SIC Code. It goes up to 10 digits, but 4 digits is precise enough for most people. The first 2 digits will give a general classification, such as 20 for the food industry, for example, and the next two digits get fairly specific, so that 2092, for example, would include companies that process fresh and frozen seafood.

The 4-digit Code is reprinted at the front of some directories, including Dun & Bradstreet's *Million Dollar Directory,* available in most libraries.

An Article on Industry Trends
Can Give You Instant Credibility

If you want to go beyond research, some clients have found they can impress prospective employers by writing a paper that would be suitable as an article for a trade magazine, focusing on what they see as emerging trends or some other interesting subject related to the industry they are targeting. In some cases, they even contact editors to see if they can get it published.

Whether they can or not, they can still send the paper along with a letter to a decision-maker at an employer prospect, saying they hope to have it published soon, but wanted to share it with the employer for two reasons. It might contain some helpful ideas for the employer, and selfishly, they'd like to put some of those ideas to work as an employee for the organization.

The existence of the article, you see, immediately changes the employer's perspective from *"Aren't you rusty?"* to *"Can we use the talents of this person who obviously is a well informed forward thinker, and understands the significance of our industry's trends?"* It doesn't guarantee you'll get an interview, but it sure solves the problem of people thinking you might be rusty.

A Speculative Presentation

And just as you can write an article, you can do "speculative work" in your field. A computer programmer, for example, can show or discuss some of the software he or she has developed while on disability. An information systems designer can do the same for systems developed for particular applications. A salesman of medical equipment can show some of the approaches he would use for recently introduced products.

Trading Free Services for Current Experience

You may even choose to contact someone in your industry or profession, and work with or for them at no charge, in order to bring yourself up-to-date and establish some momentum.

A client of mine in the midwest, a lawyer, recently did that, offering to work in the offices of another lawyer for relatively little compensation. It has given him a psychological lift to be productive, have an office to go to, and earn at least some money while he searches for a permanent position.

An alternative to free services is to work at a reduced salary for some period. If you do that, check to see if your insuror might be willing to supplement your salary for a short period of trial employment.

"Can you handle this job physically?"

A fourth problem that is common for people on disability is the basic question, *"Are you physically able to handle this work?"* One of the knowledgeable professionals in the industry who were kind enough to read a draft of this book and give me feedback, pointed out that under the Americans With Disabilities Act, the EEOC advises employers, after describing job tasks or essential functions, to ask the question this way: *"Are you able to perform these tasks with or without an accommodation?"*

Legal considerations aside, and whether an employer is genuinely interested in hiring you or looking for an excuse not to, the accurate answer in most situations probably is:

"With a few simple and relatively inexpensive modifications to

the workplace, I have absolutely no physical limitations that would prevent me from performing well in this position."

The key here is to think creatively. If you can't sit or stand for long periods, how difficult is it to have a work station with an adjustable-height table that can be easily raised or lowered, allowing you to do your work sitting or standing? Specially designed chairs and stools are commonplace today, and many of them help lessen pain and increase the amount of time you can sit. Here's another area where your insuror may be willing to step in and help out with the costs involved, and they may even provide creative suggestions, either directly or through a vendor.

Time and Technology are On Your Side

Technology here is truly your greatest ally. Advances are being made so quickly in so many areas, that circumstances you might have been resigned to just a few years ago need no longer be tolerated. It's up to you, of course, to take the initiative and keep yourself informed of any and all developments that may affect your condition or make your disability less of a barrier to productive work, whether you work for yourself at home, or for an employer.

Here are three recent examples. One of my clients who lives in Louisiana had three back operations and one neck operation. He was constantly in pain, at a level intense enough that required fairly strong drugs to get through it. The combination of fighting the pain and taking the drugs left him with only about 2 or 3 good hours per day, where he could focus his mind sharply.

He's a brilliant fellow who had designed and implemented

complex information and control systems to coordinate activities on major construction projects, and we had developed some promising opportunities for him to return to gainful employment. The limit of 2 to 3 "good" hours per day, however, made them impractical.

The solution in his case was a combination of things. He identified a particular chair that helped a lot. He found a new physical therapist whose approach resulted in less pain. And he discovered an emerging sound technology, dubbed bio-acoustics, that lessened the level of pain he felt, enabling him to reduce his drug intake.

The overall results? More energy and stamina, and an ability to work effectively for 5 to 6 hours each day, instead of 2 or 3. He started a small consulting business, has considered joining a veterinarian in a business that tracks dog licenses for the city in which he lives, and has been approached by his old employer to work on special projects.

Here's a different kind of example about technology. A client in the Southwest had been a key operating executive for a high-tech company in robotics. When he suddenly became legally blind, he could no longer keep up-to-date on the latest developments in six technologies, a requirement for him to function properly. This inability to absorb a lot of information appeared to be a significant obstacle in identifying new opportunioties for him.

Fortunately, scanner/synthesizer technology that cost $35,000 three or four years ago, now is available for $5500. He can now place any printed or typed material on a portable machine that will read it to him at greatly speeded up rates, and can absorb some types of information aurally almost as well as he could visually.

In practical terms, where he had previously been extremely

limited, this technology allows him to work with venture capital firms, some leading scientific institutions, and some private companies, to accelerate the development of selected technologies and find new applications for them.

For two other clients, one an accountant and one a medical doctor, both of whom had to face a strenuous course of study and exams, and both of whom suffered from problems with concentration and short-term memory, some inexpensive sound tapes helped them get through successfully. The tapes are based on a technology that apparently helps bring the two hemispheres of the brain into synchronization, thereby aiding concentration.

Medical Developments Are On Your Side

There are many positive medical developments as well. One, for example, could have positive implications for people recovering from a stroke or accident. In experiments on the brain and nervous system, teams of scientists and physicians have discovered that individual cells are able to communicate among themselves in previously unsuspected ways. By introducing alternate sets of signals to the brain, which can apparently be initiated by something as simple as body movements and visualization, they have learned that the brain and nervous system are quite dynamic.

Their experiments indicate that *apparently the brain and nervous system can build alternate circuits with different sets of signals, to create new connections.* They've termed it "neuroplasticity." The implications are that recovery from strokes and accidents does not necessarily have to be limited to levels previously accepted as normal, *and that there is indeed a scientific basis for what used to be termed "miracle cures."*

The implications of technological advances are not limited just to physical disabilities either. One of my clients in Texas had been suffering from depression, but apparently had made a dramatically fast recovery, to the point where his doctors felt he was ready to start working with me.

He told me jokingly that electric shock therapy had been the answer, then explained the science had developed to the point where doctors now administer just tiny amounts of current that go directly to various receptors in the brain. The term for it now is apparently *cranial electrostimulation,* and in his case, he says, it made a powerful and positive difference.

And in addition to conventional medical developments,

there is apparently a growing awareness on the part of medical doctors that some people may play a far greater role in their own recovery than previously suspected, through visualization and other means. The fast-reading book *Remarkable Recovery,* by Caryle Hirshberg and Marc Ian Barasch, gives many examples of people who surprised their doctors by recovering from a serious illness. The implication of their findings is that closer study of this phenomenon by the medical community may one day result in their identifying specific things people can do on their own, to enhance their chances for recovery from serious illness.

Closing Thoughts on Potential Employer Concerns

Whatever concerns you may have, or whatever objections you may anticipate from employers, rest assured there is most likely a way to neutralize most of them or turn them to advantage. Sometimes that requires actions before you get into interviews, and at other times they can be handled during interviews. Either way, the key to turning them around always starts with you, and your own belief that they can indeed be turned to your advantage.

A lot of what has been said here for people seeking jobs can also apply for people who intend to go into business. The difference is that, instead of impressing employers, they may need to impress potential investors, creditors, suppliers or partners.

For many people, the option of going into business is the option of choice, in some cases out of necessity, but for others simply because it provides a lot of advantages. We'll take a look at that option in Chapter 8. Before we do, we'll consider next the benefits -- and pure joy -- of getting into action.

7.

ACTION ..... THE ANTIDOTE TO ISOLATION AND
The Key to The Opportunity Collision

So far we've talked a lot about thinking, preparing, and adopting certain perspectives in your mind. While it's true that the most important work is done there, it is of no avail until you *get into action.* As I told one client recently, after he told me that God would send him an opportunity at the right time, God might also expect that he'd be out there doing all he could to catch the opportunity when it is sent. And the way to do that is to get into action, doing all you can each day to uncover opportunities.

There are so many wonderful things about taking action! Probably the best is, *action displaces fear!* When the World War II hero, Audie Murphy, was asked if he was afraid when he charged enemy trenches with a grenade in his hand, his answer was worth remembering. He was actually shaking with fear, he said, up to the moment when he pulled the pin on the grenade and started running toward the enemy.

At that moment, he explained, as soon as he got into action, there just wasn't any room for fear. He didn't have to think about or fight the fear. Quite simply, he was preoccupied with taking action, and there was no room in his mind, no time, and no place inside him, that he had left over for fear. In his opinion, you can't be acting and fearing at the same time, even if you wanted to.

Action *displaces* fear, he said, just as when you put a ship in water, it displaces the water. The ship and the water can't be in the same place at the same time, and so it is with action and fear.

Now if you substitute for *fear* the word *anxiety,* or *doubt,* or *immobility,* or *inertia,* the same principle applies. If any of those have crowded your mind or clouded your spirits, know that part of the answer to achieving peace of mind and feeling a sense of progress is to get into action.

Another positive is that acting *gets you past indecision.* It's almost a cliche for people faced with a problem to say, "Let's get past this thing," or "Let's get this behind us." The one sure way to stop worrying about whether you are going to make the right decision, and to get a problem or challenge behind you, is to *act* on it.

Still another positive ..... action *feels good!* Think about any time in your life when you were taking action on something you cared about or enjoyed. Maybe it was helping someone else, building something, planting a shrub or garden, learning to ride a bike, taking a stand on a controversial issue, or taking steps in your job that improved efficiency and productivity.

Can you remember how it felt at those moments when you were taking those actions? Maybe you'd thought about them for some time, without much feeling. But when you started acting, *it felt good,* didn't it?

One of the happiest things about getting into action can be especially significant for anyone with a disability. One of the common problems for my clients, they tell me, is that they gradually become isolated from people, and miss the interaction they used to have with friends and people they met during the course of their work day.

Almost by definition, *action means interacting with other*

people, and as that happens, bit by bit, the isolation grows less rigid, and you begin to feel a greater connectedness with others. Action also *creates its own energy force,* and you can feel yourself uniting with others in spirit. You can feel the combined energies of your action and theirs. The math always works out so that 1+1 always equals more than 2, in some cases substantially more.

If you want to win a job offer or get a business started, the single most important thing about action is, it's *The Key to The Opportunity Collision.* There's a world out there right now, where a lot of things are happening, a lot of businesses growing, new jobs being created, thousands of people realizing they're going to need a good person for something or other ..... but none of that has a chance of touching your life if you're not out there *acting.*

If it is not one of the universal laws of nature, then it should be classified as a most-of-the-time law of nature, that people who are actively seeking a specific type of opportunity will, in the course of their efforts, be presented with *at least one opportunity they never expected and weren't looking for.* I've based that "law" on the experiences of my clients, and I've long since stopped being surprised when it happens.

The world becomes a much more exciting place when you're out there in action. Who wants to know exactly how their life will play out for years ahead? That's boring. Secure maybe, but very boring. When you're out there in the path of opportunity, any day, at any moment, in almost any place, it can seem to come out of nowhere and sideswipe you when you're not looking. How exciting! All you need to do is to stay in action, and keep your mind open to lots of good things happening to you and for you.

For a job search, I recommend to my clients that they use

each of the four basic *action* avenues geared toward uncovering opportunities. For the most part, they apply also to people who want to start or purchase a business. They are reviewed briefly here.

Action Avenue #1 ..... Me-Directed Contacts

These are actions you can take based on who you are, what your interests and activities are, who you know, and who you can get to know. It is often referred to as networking, and most people don't do it very well. They ask in an informal manner for something that's almost impossible. Their chances for positive results will increase if instead they ask in a structured manner for something that's very possible.

Most people will casually approach a friend, let's call him Joe, and ask, "Joe, do you know of any openings?" Chances are, Joe doesn't, but he wants to help his friend, and says, "No, but I'll sure keep my eyes and ears open, and let you know if I hear of anything. Be sure to use me as a reference whenever you think it might help."

Joe feels bad that he can't help his friend. It's not pleasant to dwell on what you can't do for your friend, when that friend could really use your help. It's painful. So about 20 seconds after lending verbal encouragement, Joe stops thinking seriously about it.

Far better for you and Joe if the request goes like this:

"Joe, I'm looking for a new job. I want to go over my resume with you, and tell you the kinds of positions I'm going after. It's unlikely you'd know of anything, and I don't really expect that you could introduce me to someone who can make a job offer. You can still help me though.

"Could you take some time over the next few days to think about who you know? Each of us knows people the other doesn't. You may know some people who get around a lot and hear of things. One of them might know someone who knows someone who knows the person who could offer me a job. You never know where a series of referrals will lead.

"So maybe you can think of someone in sales or real estate, someone who works in a bank, an accountant, a lawyer, or some people who run businesses in the area. For all I know, you might even know a mechanic out at the airport who services planes for all the business owners who fly out of here. I'm not sure who you might think of, but I sure appreciate your giving it some thought, and I'll get back in touch early next week.

"I can't thank you enough, and remember, I'm not expecting that you'll know anyone who can offer a job directly. Talk to you next week."

Joe now feels good that he can help his friend, and he keeps on thinking. Chances are, he'll come up with at least a few names. Now you may think works only for mid- and entry-level jobs. Not so. Using this approach, a client in the midwest, a fellow who knows how to turn around manufacturing companies, started with just three personal contacts, and in three months was able to sit down for a meaningful discussion with over 100 people. About 25% of them were in positions where they could make a strong referral to someone in a position to make a hiring decision.

Following up regularly with people, and letting them know about your progress, can often help keep you in the forefront of their thinking, and stimulate them to think about new contacts for you. Remember, the world changes every day, and new opportunities are always arising.

Now if you don't have a lot of personal contacts to start with, if you've recently moved to a new location, for example, that doesn't mean you can't use this avenue effectively. That's because you can also make contacts with *people you don't know now, but can get to know.* If any of them help you, they become your friends, so I call them *future friends.*

Who are they? Almost anybody. In almost any area, for example, there will be real estate agents who often know a lot about businesses moving into the area, accountants who handle taxes for many local companies, bankers, local politicians, members of service clubs and the Chamber of Commerce, and someone who's responsible for attracting new businesses into the region.

There are also ministers, priests and rabbis, local college placement offices, building contractors, insurance brokers, and stock brokers. Be sure to think about your interests and talents as well. Are there local clubs or groups formed around an interest or hobby that appeals to you? Is there a local chapter of a national association connected with your industry or profession?

When you contact these people, you have an essential part of human nature working for you. Almost anyone feels good when they are able to help another person, and if someone can help you just by thinking of a few names, they are usually more than happy to do so. You may be surprised at the number of people who are able and willing to provide a name or two.

When they do, you proceed just as you would with people you already know. Ask for names, not job offers, and be sure to follow up with them.

Action Avenue #2 ..... Event-Directed Contacts

Every day, in almost every organization, events happen. Most of the time, they are not a signal that a job might be created there soon. But sometimes they are. And when they are, those events can make news. A company might sign a lease on office space, or announce the opening of a new branch or location. There might be a promotion or reorganization.

Perhaps someone in a company makes a speech that mentions some of the toughest problems they are facing. Or you might read about a new product being offered, or a division of a company being spun off as an independent operation. You might see ads run by a company staffing up in functions different from your own, indicating they might need to staff up in your function as well.

Whether the news is good, bad, or indifferent, it may be a signal of an emerging opportunity. So it will help you to put a filter in your mind, and ask yourself for every piece of information that comes your way, "Does this perhaps signal some kind of opportunity for me?"

Use "falling domino thinking," and imagine all the potential implications of that event, not just on the company itself, but also on its customers, suppliers and competitors.

But you don't need to limit yourself to just passively screening information that happens to come your way. You can also go out and *make events happen,* and intentionally be where the action is. You can take the initiative to attend conferences and shows, develop your own product ideas or advertising campaign on speculation, or write a paper that highlights important industry trends, which you send to decision makers and/or to editors of trade magazines.

For the "passive" mode, where you see an event in the

news, your approach is simply that you noticed it, and figured it might be a signal they'd be needing someone with your talents. The method of contact doesn't matter. You can write a letter, phone, or go in person. Regardless, when you use this avenue you often enjoy substantial advantages. The employer will surely be impressed that you were smart enough to figure out an opportunity might be emerging, and took the initiative to contact them.

You've obviously exhibited a lot of enthusiasm. And if they are thinking about hiring someone, there's a chance for you to get in there and win the job before it "goes public" through an ad or recruiter. Instead of 50 competitors for the job, you may be the only one considered.

For the "active" mode, your approach might be the same as for the "passive" mode, but you have some additional options. You can, for example, enclose a paper you've written that highlights some significant trends you anticipate, mentioning that the reader may find them interesting, and that you would be interested in working for the company. This is the same approach mentioned earlier for overcoming the problem of not having experience in a particular industry. It can also work, of course, when you *do* have experience in an industry.

Action Avenue #3 ..... Position-Directed Contacts

When a position has been advertised or placed in the hands of a recruiter, if your background comes close to fitting, it makes sense to get your resume in there with those of the other contenders.

That's also the problem, of course. When an organization has already gone to the trouble of defining and advertising a position, or is willing to pay a recruiter to find suitable candidates, they will draw up very tight specifications for the job, get a lot of responses, and it's usually a highly competitive situation.

Nevertheless, if your background might fit, you certainly want to be considered, despite the high odds. There are a few things you can do to bring down the odds. With recruiters and agencies, recognize that they are paid by employers, not applicants, and the chances of their having an assignment to get someone like you, at the moment you conact them, are pretty slim.

So you can change the odds in your favor by contacting a number of them. For senior level positions, it's not uncommon to contact 300 or more. (For local mid- or entry-level positions, the number would be much smaller.) There are directories you can refer to, with a lot of helpful general information, as well as contact information for recruiters all over the country. The best known is published by Kennedy Publishing in Fitzwilliam, New Hampshire. They also supply specialized lists and labels of recruiters.

For answering ads, don't disqualify yourself because you don't have all they are asking for. Employers seldom get the ideal person, and when they do, that person may not want the job for what they are willing to pay.

And sometimes you can persuade an employer to "upgrade" a position for which you are overqualified. You just tell them you can do all they are asking for and more, and would like to discuss the possibility of adding to the job responsibilities. You can point out that if they would be willing to pay just a little more, you'd give them an excellent return on their extra investment.

A lot of people don't follow up on ads, so if you do, whether in writing or by phone, you can sometimes give yourself an extra edge. You're showing enthusiasm, persistence, and getting your resume on top of the pile.

Last, remember, ads are sometimes signals of other emerging opportunities. They are themselves "events" that signal a company may soon be hiring in functions that are not now being advertised.

Action Avenue #4 ..... Employer-Directed Contacts

In this action avenue, you identify employers who are your most logical targets, those most likely to need someone with your talents. Usually you do this by deciding on the the types of employers by line of business or industry, their sizes, and locations.

You then write, call or visit a decision maker in your function, who would probably be the person you report to, or that person's boss. In your letter you briefly get across your "selling proposition," or the reason why they would want to hire you, and promise to follow up by phone within a week.

You normally need to contact a number of employers, sometimes 100 or more, in order to find one or two who might be interested. Your letters or calls are essentially a form of research.

The logic is as follows. Every day new problems arise and new duties are created in many companies. Most of the time they are handled by people already employed, or if a new position is created, it is given to someone with a contact inside the organization.

But not always, and if you reach enough decision makers in enough companies, chances are that you'll reach one or two of them at a time when they anticipate needing someone like you within the next few months.

When that happens, and you meet the decison maker before the position actually opens up, you become the person with the "inside connection" when it is time to hire.

As with any other action avenue, followup helps to turn the odds in your favor. And whenever you can start your letter or conversation by referring to a third party who suggested you contact the company, or who might be known to the decision maker, that can often help as well.

In general, your letter or conversation should not focus so much on your strengths, as on those areas where the employer might need help, and where you can contribute. You can use a "high level of assumption" about your ability to contribute, leaving it for CARE stories and a resume to back up your claims.

(CARE stories are concise stories about challenges you handled effectively, that are similar to the challenges being faced by the prospective employer. CARE is an acronym for Challenge, Actions, Results, Experience Gained. The information-surfacing forms mentioned earlier are helpful in putting such stories together.)

Employers really aren't interested in your experience and achievements, no matter how impressive, until they first know whether and how you can help them.

So first things first, and if you're not sure where an employer might need assistance, point to those areas where you're best equipped to contribute, and state that you'd like to deliver results for them just as you have for past employers.

A Consistent Action Plan

You'll find that if you are consistently active each day in at least one of the four action avenues, you'll eventually have opportunities coming your way on a regular basis. An outline reviewing the four avenues follows on the next page.

It's important to remember, no matter how well or how poorly you implement an action plan, or whether you even have a plan, for that matter, there is an infinite difference between inaction and action. As soon as you start to act, no matter how effectively, you will begin to enjoy all the advantages mentioned at the beginning of this chapter.

So do it!

The Four Action Avenues For Uncovering Opportunities

#1 Me-Directed Contacts

"Present Friends" _Family _Professors _Fellow Participants in civic, social, political, religious, or political activities _Neighbors _Classmates _Community _Customers _Suppliers _People you reported to, or who reported to you, or worked with you _Salespeople or professionals you've been a customer for (car, insurance, travel, banker, lawyer, real estate, investments, instructor, boat, clothing, accountant).

"Future Friends" _People with similar interests, hobbies, circumstances _People now holding the kind of job you want _People now running the kind of business you're interested in _People whose information, contacts or influence may be helpful ... _Editors and publishers _Association Officials _Elected Officials _Consultants _Bankers, accountants and lawyers _Business Owners _Board members _University Deans

_Economic development officials _Local religious leaders _Trustees

_Athletic coaches _Real estate agents _Chamber of Commerce

#2 Event-Directed Contacts

Active: Attend meetings, join societies, write papers, etc.

Passive: (news) Growth companies, new products, expansion, relocation, promotions, new technologies, excerpts of speeches, etc.

#3 Position-Directed Contacts

Ads: Identified by position descriptions

Recruiters: Identified by specialty, income level, location

#4 Employer-Directed Contacts

One-Contact: Identified by industry, product line, service, location, size

Multi-Contact: Preferred targets, using the same criteria

Items For Preparation: _printing and word processing, _groundwork with references, _interview (CARE stories, handling liabilities, answering questions, selling techniques), _ lists of friends and "future friends," _reading to gain credibility _mental conditioning _uncompensated service to gain current experience, _physical condition and appearance

8.
DO YOU WANT TO GO INTO BUSINESS?

Eight years ago, only about 20% of my clients wanted to go into business. Most still preferred to find a job. Recently, the percentage preferring to start or purchase a business has climbed substantially. That may reflect the way Vocational Rehabilitation Coordinators view my services, in that they tend to think of me for people who want to start or purchase a business. But there are probably other reasons. Much of that time period was one of recession, so jobs were tougher to find. And despite the Americans With Disabilities Act, most people on disability believe they are at a serious disadvantage when it comes to getting hired.

Some know that they cannot be reliable employees, and would have difficulty with a regular schedule, either because of pain, lack of mobility, lack of stamina, or some combination of those factors. Whatever the factors that may make going into business a *necessity,* many consider that there are a number of advantages even if it is not a necessity, but rather, an *option.*

There is first of all the satisfaction of "being your own boss," It also gives you a good deal of freedom and flexibility. You can be as versatile as you like. And if you need to take a nap or lie down for certain periods during the workday, no one is going to think it's odd, or make a disparaging comment to the boss.

And when you're in business for yourself, you are usually

doing what you love to do, or you wouldn't be in the business. So there's the element of pure personal enjoyment.

Just as important for many people is the opportunity for significant earnings. Often disability has caused financial problems, and a person's entire family has had to drastically scale back its style of living. If a business has enough potential, it may hold the promise of generating pre-disability earnings levels, or exceeding them.

Some of my clients are seasoned business executives who have managed large organizations. They need little or no help in evaluating opportunities and getting their businesses started. Others are not so seasoned, but nonetheless have options for starting or buying simpler businesses that look appealing to them.

For those clients I've developed my "going into business" forms, which pose eight basic questions that anyone contemplating a business might do well to ask themselves. In the instructions for those forms, there are some guidelines and helpful thoughts, which are reprinted on ten pages at the back of this book. If you're not experienced in writing plans or making financial projections, you may want to enlist the aid of friends who are.

"Settling" Your Claim

Clients interested in starting a business sometimes ask the insuror to "settle" their policies, in order to get the capital required. "Settling" usually means that they receive a sum of money from the insuror, and in return they give up any claims they may have to benefits under the policy. Sometimes the "settlement" will be structured in such a way that the person doesn't get all cash, but a combination of cash and an annuity, for example, to provide some element of security.

In the event that a "settlement" might be of interest to you, I'll put down a few thoughts here that might prove helpful. This is an area where there is a lot of misunderstanding, and there tends to be an element of mystery about it. There are many elements of it that remain a mystery to me, so the points here will be made only briefly, and in general terms.

First, some insurors will not consider settlements. Among those that will, they might be open to settlement at one point in time, but have no interest at another time. Insurors are not obliged to settle a claim when requested to do so. They can if they choose just keep paying your monthly benefit.

While insurors are not obliged to settle a long term disability claim, they can be positively disposed to do so, if it can be shown that it would be beneficial to the claimant and to themselves. When insurors are happy to settle, it is usually because they can be reasonably assured it will be financially beneficial to the claimant, and because they will "free up reserves" and get some liabilities off their books by doing so.

For example, if they are paying you $3000 per month until age 65, and you are 45, then theoretically they could be paying you $36,000 for 20 years, or a total of $720,000. A lot of people mistakenly think, if they settle, that's the amount they should get.

Insurors don't see it that way, however. The people who determine what you'll be offered are not those in Vocational Rehabilitation, but rather, people on the financial side. They use various calculations that result in their putting a certain amount of money into reserves for paying that claim. You might think it would be simply the amount of money they would need to put into safe investments, in order to generate enough money to pay your claim each month, but it's not that simple.

Using complex calculations, they figure out formulas and multipliers for certain categories, and if your case falls in one of them, there isn't much you can do about it, as I understand it. The amount you'd be offered would be smaller, for example, if you fall in a category where most people go back to work in a few years, or are likely to recover from the disability. And depending on the nature of your disability and the terms of your policy, there may be varying degrees of probability as to whether you will still qualify for benefits after certain periods.

As you can see, it's an area that is anything but clearcut, but if you request a settlement and if it makes sense from the insuror's standpoint (often it doesn't), they are likely to get back with an offer. The problem is, it is difficult to know what an insuror will offer you. I'm often surprised. Don't be shocked if the offer is 30% or less of what you'd get if you received benefit payments over the full term of the policy, and don't be surprised if the offer is not open to negotiation. Occasionally it might be, but many times it's not.

With one exception, I have no advice here, but I do have an observation. It is about people who want to settle to invest in a business, but don't think the settlement offer is large enough. Some get annoyed, and withdraw their settlement request. Others also get annoyed, but calculate that the offer, while not as large as they had wanted, is nevertheless large enough for them to start or buy a business that will generate the level of earnings they want, so they settle.

The one thing I'd strongly advise *against* is letting a lawyer who doesn't know much about settlements of disability policies, try to negotiate for you with the insuror. Some think they know and confuse it with settlements of Workers Compensation claims. They are not similar. In one case I worked for months with a fellow to get a food wholesaling business off the ground, with the clear understanding that any settlement would be within a certain range. Everything looked positive until, at the last moment, his lawyer demanded 10 times what the insuror was offering. The insuror withdrew the offer.

The Element of Risk

If your proposed business is risky, or if you have little business experience and no plan, and you need your benefit payments to live on, it's probably not a good idea to ask for a settlement, and you may well find the insuror is unwilling to consider one if you do ask for it. The same holds true if your health is such that there is a good chance you will have to cut back your involvement substantially, before you get it to the point that someone else can take over for you.

Some clients who have other resources, and do not need their benefit payments to live on, are quite happy to take their chances, even in a risky business. For those who depend even partially on benefits to meet their living expenses, however, it is well to remember that if your business fails, you are left with no income from the business and no benefit payments. And if the business is not generating income, it's not likely to be worth very much if you attempt to sell it.

A number of clients have told me that they can't rely on benefits for the long term, because they are depleting their savings, and need to find a business that will generate more income than the benefits are providing. It's evident they need to do something, and operating a business is sometimes their most realistic option. If you are faced with that set of circumstances, then it pays to minimize your risks to the greatest extent possible.

If you are determined to go into business, one way to minimize risk is to purchase an existing business that has a track record of stable earnings over a period of years. If it is not a business that depends for its success on the personal charisma, contacts, or skills of the current owner, and if you can determine that no significant changes will happen after you buy, such as a rent increase, a nearby construction project, the closing of a nearby factory or office park, a sudden increase in the number of competitors, or a change in the buying habits of your customers, then you'll obviously have less risk than you would if any of these were about to happen.

You also need to objectively assess your own abilities and determination, as they relate to the current owner. Is that person a super sales personality? Are you? Does the current owner work 16 hours a day? Can you, and do you expect to? Will you need to make a number of changes in the way the business is currently operated? How do you know those changes will affect profits favorably?

Another way some clients purchasing businesses have minimized risk is to pay a certain percentage down, then get the current owner to agree that the balance due will go up or down depending upon profit levels. This gives the current owner an incentive to help you become successful.

The Benefits of Accounting and Legal Advice, and a Plan

Tax laws change, of course, and so do interpretations, but there are tax-wise ways to purchase a business. For example, in some instances people have structured purchase agreements in a way that minimizes the seller's capital gains taxes and spreads the seller's income over a number of years. The buyer can then request, in view of the tax savings, that the seller lower the asking price. Whether you are buying a business or just its assets, it's advisable to check tax considerations with an accountant and lawyer, and to work closely with them in negotiating the terms of purchase.

One last point. Whether you are buying a business or starting one, you are well advised to have at least a simple plan, to help avoid unpleasant surprises, and to have a reasonable estimate ahead of time how long it will be before the business generates enough cash to support you.

9.
SOME PEOPLE WHO'VE GOTTEN JOBS,
And Taught Me About .....

In this and the following chapters, I'll share some stories about people I've had the pleasure to work with over the past 8 years, as they did what they had to do in order to get back to meaningful and productive work. Their names and some details are changed to protect their identities. The headlines before their stories summarize the main thing they taught me through their experiences and the way they acted to turn seemingly negative events into something positive. I'll start with one who taught me about .....

Visualizing ..... and Learning to be a Gracious Receiver

Tim G remains one of my favorites. A Sales Manager for a publishing company in his late 30s, he had relocated from Maryland to Colorado after learning he had multiple sclerosis. At one point before I was asked to work with him, he had decided that his physical problems were just too much, and he told his wife she might be better off to leave him because he was giving up and would probably die before too long.

In her strong, quiet way, she read him the riot act. Every day, she reminded him, she makes the decision to either stay or leave, which is always an option. She hadn't married a quitter, and if that now became his choice, she might just decide one day to leave. But for now, for today, she was staying, and asked him to return the favor by deciding to make up his mind to improve, physically and emotionally.

That turned him around. They decided he should attend a 2-week camp in the northwest run by a stern, 80-year-old European lady who was so agile she could dance like a 30-year-old. Her camp was geared to help people like Tim, who had lost most of their physical mobility, to learn a dozen basic exercises that would improve their physical conditioning.

On the first day, they placed him on the mats, but he couldn't even bend his leg to get into position to do the first exercise. The woman instructed her assistants to place him on the side of the mats, then continued with the other participants. After she was finished, she walked to the side, stood directly over him with one leg on each side, pointing her finger in his face, and told him in an authoritative tone, "You .... tonight you visualize yourself bending your leg."

As it turns out, Tim's wife was a big believer in visualization, and had apparently used it to good advantage in her life, so he assured this woman, as he lay there looking up at her, that he knew how effective visualization could be, and would certainly follow her instructions. In his heart though, as he later told me, he was greatly discouraged and didn't really believe it would help him. He was lying in bed that night thinking how easy it would be to just give up, when he thought of his wife and decided that he didn't have anything to lose by at least trying.

So until he fell asleep he lay there visualizing himself bending his leg. But he didn't believe it would work, and felt the same way in the morning, experiencing a sense of despair and hopelessness as they once again placed him on the mat. A few minutes later, much to his own amazement, on command from the 30-year-old 80-year-old, he was able to bend his leg. That filled him with such excitement that during those two weeks he quickly progressed through the basic exercises, and in another two weeks after returning from the camp he had mastered all twelve.

Shortly after that he began a two-year course in computer programming, but by the time he completed it, there was no market for programmers in his area, so the Vocational Rehabilitation Coordinator asked me to help him find another way to make a living. By this time he was getting around with a walker and a wheelchair, which he could take in and out of his specially equipped van, and had an office setup in his basement. He figured he might have enough energy and stamina to be able to get out of the office for 1/2 day per week.

He didn't have any clear idea of what he might do, however, since he'd have to work primarily from home. After reviewing his achievements on my forms, which are designed to identify the action steps people used in the past to achieve results, and after experiencing his upbeat personality over the phone, it became apparent to me that, theoretically at least, he had a number of talents that could be valuable to different types of businesses.

For salespeople on the road, he could function as a customer service person, providing in-house sales support and followup. For any small business, or for one just getting started, he could set up their administrative systems, keep their records, and help plan their marketing, advertising, promotion, and sales activities. He could also help them select their computer and software purchases, and get that system up and working.

I created a simple one-page summary of the services he could offer, and some prototype letters he could send to various types of prospects, who were identified through a computer search, combined with some local directories. When I visited with him, we rehearsed different types of sales situations he'd face over the phone and in person. Until he saw the summary and letters, and rehearsed what he'd be saying to prospects, he didn't really believe it was feasible for him to either sell or deliver those services.

But he had to admit that all the things he saw in writing were based on information he himself had provided in my forms. And the action plan we set up for selling those services made plenty of allowance for his limited mobility, energy, and stamina. So suddenly, he had everything he needed to get into action as an independent consultant. The only thing that could hold him back would be his own beliefs in limits.

Within two months he was functioning as a sales followup / customer service person for an independent distributor of heavy machinery who traveled most of the time. He had also gotten three other clients, small businesses in his area that needed administrative and sales-related help as they expanded. This small but very fast start, due primarily to his winning sales personality, brought some other forces into play.

He was so encouraged by this activity that he seemed to have more energy than he had anticipated, and was able to spend two half-days per week outside the home, not just one. He developed more confidence. This led to his contacting a lot of people, including many new prospects and a number of old business associates he hadn't been in touch with for some time. This led in short order to *The Opportunity Collision*.

An ex-boss told him of another publisher who could probably use his sales followup services in Colorado, and offered to forward his single-page summary of services to that publisher with a note of recommendation. A week later he got a call from that publisher, and within a few more weeks he was their exclusive representative in Colorado, which occupied all his available working hours.

Technically he was still an independent, but in substance he had won what amounted to a full-time job. The truly remarkable thing here is that the MS remained in remission, his energy level continued to increase, and within two years Tim was the rep for three states, taking 3-day trips in his van. One of the keys, he told me, was *Learning To Be A Gracious Receiver.*

Where previously he would never let anyone help him, now he would not hesitate to ask maintenance people who came to know him at the schools and offices he visited, or just plain passersby, to hold a door or give him a boost. A few of them told him he'd made their day, but they didn't have to say it. The positive look on their faces was testimony enough to the truth that when you let others help you, you give them a great gift.

Once he understood that, and overcame what he termed pride and stubbornness that kept him from using a wheelchair as often as he might, he found he could cover a lot more territory with a lot less energy expended. And make a lot of people happy in the process.

Patience and Perseverance

Karen B had been on disability for five years when our paths crossed. Back problems resulting from an accident had made it impossible for her to continue in the public relations job in southern California that she enjoyed so much.

The enforced idleness for such a long period had taken its toll on the spirits of this talented woman in her late 30s, but she clung to the hope that somehow she could get back to work, even with the limits on sitting, standing, bending and carrying that she had to endure. So she asked her insuror if they could provide some help in a return-to-work effort..

It was apparent from the start that Karen was very intelligent, with outstanding communications skills. What wasn't apparent until later, was a strong character, an ability to endure disappointments and never give up, that would severely try the most steadfast personality, and remains impressive by any measure.

Karen's talents were abundant enough, and her experience broad enough, that it made sense to create four separate resumes for her, one for sales, another for marketing, still another for public relations, and a fourth for journalism. It's unusual that my clients will do well by answering ads, but because her experience was strong, her resumes well written, and she made such an excellent personal impression, she did quite well.

Within two months, she had interviewed for eight positions, and implemented extremely well the interviewing techniques she learned in our personal meeting. Three situations looked promising, one in sales, one in marketing, and one in public relations. For a number of reasons, she chose the opportunity in sales, with a growing company in the health services field.

The woman who hired her had just been hired herself by the President to fill the Sales Manager post, and in good faith spelled out for her the environment in which she'd work and the opportunities available for those who performed well. It sounded ideal, and it was.

Problem was, as sometimes happens in companies undergoing a lot of change, there was an internal political struggle which the President lost, and things changed, but not until Karen had been there long enough so that she was no longer on disability payments. Now she had no disability payments and no job. Enter true grit. She wasted no time feeling sorry for herself, took part-time positions to survive financially, and revved up her job search again.

Some clients will stay in touch even though the insurors no longer retain me to assist them, and Karen asked me to continue providing some guidance, which I'm happy to do. To make a long story short, over the past four years she has landed and lost three jobs, although employers will be quick to point out she was an excellent performer. In one case she lost the job after being recruited there from another position.

But she has never lost her spirit. She's human, so it has sagged at times, but she's never lost it. Her employers have included a law firm, an accounting firm, and a public relations firm, where she has filled marketing and business development posts, and met or exceeded goals, but the combination of internal politics a few levels above her, and a poor California economy, prevented any of those from developing into long term situations.

She recently moved back to the midwest, and based on her latest input, chances are she'll soon win a desirable position there. Yes, she still has back problems and some pain, but she hasn't let that stop her. She's living testimony to the power of perseverance in the face of adversity.

Keeping Your Eye on the Goal, Not on the Pain

Debbie B, in her early 30s, lives in Manhattan. Like a number of people I work with, she had more than one disabling condition. The official cause of her disability was severe colitis, but she also had an unusual eye disease that required surgery, and suffered from hypoglycemia. At one time during our work together she traveled to Europe for special treatment of the eye disease. The colitis could be very painful, making it impractical to get anything accomplished on the "bad days."

She had worked in the Human Resources department of a major consulting firm, where she had routinely put in 50- and 60-hour weeks, and enjoyed it. But that was no longer possible. After she returned my forms, I was able to construct a resume that did not over-identify her with Human Resources, but instead positioned her for a broad range of positions within a service firm. She could use her old resume for Human Resources positions.

Despite a number of "bad" days physically, Debbie maintained her upbeat outlook and her determination to find a job she could handle without setting off colitis problems. Our first priority was to find a part-time position, for which her physician had cleared her. She was confident that if she found a challenging job in the right environment, her improved mental state would help improve her health.

In a similar circumstance, in the face of that much pain, I doubt I'd have the same level of determination, and maybe that has something to do with the fact that the people who have these disabilities seem to have a great deal more internal strength than the average person. Maybe it's born out of necessity. I don't know. I do know that, after she returned to the U. S. from a European trip where no significant progress had been made on her eye disease, she redoubled her efforts in the job search.

And within a matter of weeks she was successful. She won a Manhattan-based position with the headquarters staff of a major pharmaceutical firm, in which she could fill a number of functions. The environment, salary level and hours were precisely what we were looking for, and there was opportunity for advancement in the future.

As is the case with many clients, we never met personally, but established close rapport over the phone. This remarkable young woman wrote me a note of thanks, saying I had helped her build confidence and maintain a positive focus, but I know she did it herself. It's typical of many of my clients that they will give me and others more credit than we deserve.

On the other hand, there may be truth in what Leo Buscaglia says in his book *Born For Love,* about the many opportunities we have to make our love felt, and that too often we underestimate the power of a kind word, a listening ear, or the smallest act of caring.

Trying Again, And Again, And Again ..... and One More Time

Don S's disability involved depressed cardiac and lung functions, and put limits on his energy and stamina, but not so much that this midwesterner couldn't learn computer programming after his disability. He had previously achieved a lot in engineering as a Project Manager for an automotive parts company, but returning to that kind of demanding position was no longer feasible.

Instead, while working part-time as a computer operator, he had been trying for three years to get a job as a computer programmer, but without success. He had done a number of imaginative things, and wasn't sure there was much more he could do. He'd had so many disappointments that he was beginning to think he'd be trapped in his current dead-end position.

Fortunately I was able to put together a resume that, for the first time, presented the combination of his engineering experience, computer experience, and education in a way that made it obvious he was qualified for far more than an entry level position. This lifted his spirits, gave him a lot more confidence, and prompted him to take up once again his job search efforts. The fact that somebody else cared, didn't hurt either.

But he lived in an area with relatively few opportunities and the going was rough. When he was about to lose hope again, he got a call from an employer who had rejected him for a position before I had started to work with him.

During our work together he'd learned to develop a mindset that kept him open to nurturing anything that sounded even remotely like an opportunity. He put that to good use with this employer, and within a week of the call had gotten an offer for what we agreed was an ideal position in many respects. He would be a programmer in a small software firm where he would be an important performer for them, while he would learn those aspects of programming he still needed to master.

Three years is a long time to spend in a job that isn't challenging. It's a long time to be looking for something better, without success. No one would have blamed Don for giving up. I'm personally happy he didn't. Like Debbie, he insisted on giving me credit for building his confidence and helping him remain open to opportunity, but like Debbie, he did 99% of it himself. He got in touch afterward to let me know it was going well. Then he got in touch still later to let me know it wasn't. I helped a little. And he moved again to a still better job.

Jerry C

Another tale of perseverance, which also underscores the value of a supportive spouse, is that of Jerry C. I won't even admit how long I worked with him, but he was my longest running client. Jerry's disability was chronic fatigue syndrome, and he lived in New Hampshire, during a period in which that state led the nation in terms of worst economic depression. That's one reason why it took him so long to land a job.

He's a dedicated fellow in his 30s, and he worked very hard. Many times he came close, but never quite scored. His background was in financial operations, and he came close not only in that field, but in retailing, insurance, food processing, and other types of businesses. His disappointment at not winning these jobs was tempered somewhat when he learned, as he often did, that the company which rejected him had gone out of business shortly afterward. New Hampshire was that bad at the time.

But he persevered, and was able to stay afloat financially because his wife managed to not only keep her job at a large catering firm, but to win a promotion as well. Finally he was offered a position as a member of the faculty of a business college. The only hitch was providing a number of enthusiastic references. I instructed him on how to go about doing that, and he won the job. To this day I marvel at his patience and endurance, and his ability to spring back into action after disappointments, of which there were far too many.

10.

MORE PEOPLE WHO'VE GOTTEN JOBS,
And Taught Me About .....

The Power of a Kind Word ... or a Listening Ear.

Kyle S, in his mid-40s, had been a federal government employee, with a background in security and other areas. He'd had a number of operations on his back, from which he had some continuing pain, was experiencing severe financial difficulties while trying to keep a son in college, and was trying to care for his mother, who was ill and lived in the southeast, a 6-hour drive away. He confided that he was starting to feel pretty depressed. Who wouldn't be?

Our first conversation ended up being a long one. I'm not a psychologist, but the nature of the work is such that you've got to address issues, beliefs, and assumptions that affect a client's emotions.

We talked about a number of things, including his assumption that the government wouldn't take him back, and how he might start to become active right away as a consultant working with existing firms in one of two areas - security, and securing startup funds for new and second-stage companies. He had expertise in both areas, and as it turns out, had at one time run his own business.

We had only that one long conversation, followed up by a letter from me, and then a few shorter conversations, when his case closed successfully. Whatever was said in that first conversation, I wish I knew, but somehow it had tempered his depression and helped him see things in a more positive light.

For the first time, he told me, he felt that maybe he could exert some control over his situation and change things for the better. He followed my advice about getting back to the government, and it ended up in his getting a long part-time consulting assignment, which eased his financial situation.

He also got more aggressive about soliciting startup funding projects, and secured two that looked promising. One even had a stated promise of long term employment in addition to his fees, should the financing come through. To support that business and perhaps get started in security consulting as well, he requested and got a settlement, which made sense with the stability of his additional income.

It wasn't anything I said that helped Kyle turn things around, but rather, just the fact that I was a willing ear ..... willing to listen to him sort out his own problems and decide on his own course of action. Fortunately, it was enough.

The Problems of an Overachiever With "Too Many Strengths"

Darlene L is an extraordinary lady living in New York State, a nurse who had back and bending problems. The number of things she has done incredibly well boggles the mind, including a variety of hospital positions that involved training, direct care, emergency helicopter services and others, as well as positions outside the medical field.

But she hadn't gotten offers for some jobs she wanted,

and was fearful that she was seen as overqualified by some employers, while for others her broad-based experience didn't include all the specific "specialist" elements they were looking for.

Her problem was twofold. First, she had so many achievements in so many different positions (about 12), that it was difficult to get across all her strengths without confusing the reader. But we succeeded in doing so on her resume and it impressed a lot of people, including Darlene. Second, she needed just the right words to say, so that prospective employers would feel comfortable that such a high-powered person would be happy in the position they were offering.

We hammered out the right words, and you only had to tell her once. Before she had even received my followup letter, she had used all the techniques I recommended. Next day in fact. Within 10 days of getting the new resume, she had three potential offers to consider in each of the three areas where she had an interest ..... a law firm, a hospital, and an independent emergency medical facility.

We sorted out her priorities as we discussed them, but once again, the "close encounter" with each option made her decision an easy one. She discouraged the law firm from making an offer, maintained positive relations with the hospital while turning them down, and accepted the offer from a group of doctors to manage the startup of an independent emergency facility, after we reshaped the job slightly to accommodate her situation.

Battling Discouragement When You Keep Coming In Second

Marty D from New Jersey was a salesman in his late 30s

who had been successful in selling to supermarkets for a major biscuit company. When we started to work together, he'd been out for 18 months due to a back injury. He'd also gone through a recent divorce. His resume conveyed no achievements, although he certainly had them.

Clearly, it was going to take not just a stronger resume, but also a lot of encouragement to help him build the emotional firepower he'd need to come back from these negative events. Come back he did, though, and he worked hard to implement the action plan we had designed.

In each of the four basic action avenues for uncovering job opportunities, he would do whatever was necessary. He was willing to move, and we were able to expand the number of industries where he would have credibility by highlighting selected areas of achievement, so he got a lot of response from recruiters.

Response, that is, but no interviews. Over 60 recruiters, out of 500 contacted, called him with positive feedback on the achievements in his resume and "future prospects" in their area. But not one led to an interview. That's very unusual. Recruiters usually don't call unless they have an assignment that fits you, but this was a particularly difficult time for recruiters.

Fortunately for Marty, answering ads, contacting employers directly, networking, and developing opportunities based on events, all proved to be more fruitful. He interviewed for over a dozen good jobs in six months, but each time came out second or third. His spirits sagged then, probably lower than they had a number of times before. Suddenly, as so often happens when things look bleakest, three good opportunities surfaced.

He was a finalist for all of them. At last, no more "Mr.

Second or Third." Two turned into offers, one in medical products and the other in foods. Both met our criteria for a suitable job, and both promised future growth potential, but he opted to go with the industry he knew. His back condition was not a problem for the national company that hired him.

Getting Past Doubts About Racial Discrimination ..... With Enthusiasm

Ed T remains one of my favorite clients. A former bench chemist in a southwestern state, Ed had developed back problems which caused him to go on disability. His condition had improved to the point where he had been searching for a job more than three months when he asked the insuror for assistance, and was referred to me.

Ed was a brilliant fellow, with degrees in Chemical Engineering and Math, graduate studies in Operations Management and Industrial Technology, and a solid work record. There were some problems, though. He was extremely soft-spoken and, as is true of many people with a scientific bent, not very adept at self-promotion. Also, he had decided to switch from chemist to a process engineering position, and while he had the educational credentials, didn't have experience specifically in process engineering.

Complicating matters was the fact that Ed was an Afro-American, and sometimes felt people were surprised when a black man showed up for the interview. This was beginning to get to him emotionally, since he never knew when, where, or whether this might be a problem.

We got past that quickly. Ed agreed with me that he didn't want to waste time interviewing with anyone who'd reject him on the basis of ethnic group membership, so we included in his cover letter the fact that he was Afro-American, which might be important for employers trying to meet Affirmative Action goals, but that he wanted to be hired only for his ability to contribute, not to fill a quota. No more surprises at interviews, and no more uncertainties about motivation. The resulting peace of mind helped Ed considerably.

We conducted a multi-state job search, contacting hundreds of recruiters and employers identified in a computer search. Ed had over two dozen interviews over the next three months, but while people seemed to react favorably, he didn't get any offers. We worked on ways he could express more enthusiasm in his low-key manner, and hammered out specific words he could use in followup letters, that would reinforce the enthusiasm factor.

It finally worked, and he got what he considered an ideal position, finally making the switch from chemist to process engineer. Three weeks after he'd been hired, his boss told him that they liked him originally, but not enough to hire him. It was after all three people who interviewed him got a personalized enthusiastic followup letter, that they changed their minds. In a meeting the day they got the letters, the boss had said to the other two, "How can we pass up someone who is this excited about joining us?"

Coming Oh So Close ..... and Missing

Jim V had been a highly successful medical sales rep, selling primarily to hospitals in a large midwestern city for a major medical products manufacturer, and then taking on an international marketing position, before his stroke.

He had largely recovered after two years, but wasn't having much success in a job search, and asked his insuror for some assistance. In his late 50s, he felt his age was against him, as well as the perception of some people that a stroke leaves you less capable on a permanent basis.

While he had gotten some interviews, he hadn't received any offers. The letters and resume he had prepared were just average, and didn't really get across his strong record of achievement that was evident from the information he filled out on my forms. We developed stronger materials, and an action plan that included not only local opportunities, but also contact with national firms that might want a rep to cover the region surrounding the city in which he lived.

For specific contact information, we identified a suitable directory, and Jim succeeded in developing some interest on the part of many companies, but none quite strong enough to create a new position for him. The *Opportunity Collision* came into play here, as Jim suddenly received an offer for a job he hadn't really sought, totally apart from the medical field.

He and his wife had been active for some time in church activities, helping teenagers, and now the church at the national level was interested in hiring a couple to tour a large midwest region, training the local trainers for its program aimed at helping teenagers. It didn't pay the kind of money Jim wanted, but the other satisfactions of the job outweighed that, and he had decided to accept it.

He did, and was on an emotional high in anticipation of all the good he could do, when the offer was suddenly taken away. Politics can extend even into church organizations, apparently, and another, more "connected" couple was offered the position. Jim was embarrassed, depressed, and not sure he had the motivation to keep searching.

I have a theory that when people spend a great deal of energy and emotion pursuing something, and almost but don't quite make it happen, all that energy kind of hangs around in the air somewhere, just waiting to make something else happen, so that inevitably something else does pop up very quickly, and it's likely to be every bit as appealing as the thing that didn't happen.

Theory or no, in Jim's case it happened. Within two weeks of his big disappointment, he started his job search efforts again, and one of the four action avenues (this time networking) turned up an old acquaintance. It seems this fellow had started up a medical products company in another midwest city, and needed someone with Jim's background to handle marketing and also act as National Sales Manager, signing up reps or distributors in various parts of the country.

After a few discussions, a job description was worked out that suited Jim perfectly. He'd spend one week per month in the other city, one or two weeks traveling, and one or two working from his home town. His wife could travel with him when and if she pleased.

In retrospect, Jim feels he never would have found this opportunity if he hadn't first lost the other. He's also convinced somebody "up there" is watching out for him. Maybe. And maybe it's a case of just not giving up.

11.
STILL MORE PEOPLE WHO'VE GOTTEN JOBS,
And Taught Me About .....

Searching Through The Pain, and Finding The Silver Lining

Ned was a key executive with a large retail chain, working in the Southeast, when severe colitis forced him to go on disability. He'd been out over a year when he was referred to me. He still had a lot of pain on occasion, but wanted to get started on a job search. As good an executive as he was, he hadn't really appreciated just how valuable his contributions had been, until he filled out my information-surfacing forms and saw the resume created for him, based on that information.

This renewed his confidence and enthusiasm, and letters were created showing him how he could approach people in the industry on an upbeat note, with an eye toward the future, rather than taking a defensive tone about the disability. We laid out a carefully structured plan, involving hundreds of contacts, and over ten months' time this resulted in several interviews for high-level executive positions in retail all across the country.

But nothing clicked. Despite very positive feedback

after interviews, in many instances where there were no other contenders, no offers developed. We checked out potential reference problems, and found there were none. It seemed a case of his position being so important, that it often was not just a plain hiring decision, but rather, a question of the basic direction a company was to take, and inertia usually prevailed.

Ned's physical condition took a turn for the worse at this time, developing into Crohn's Disease, causing more intense pain, and we called off our efforts for a few months. His doctors did some good things for him, and he was ready to start again, but we had noticed a correlation between the pain and the job search activity. Our conclusion? The stress of the job search exacerbated the pain. So we restricted job search efforts to contacts with friends, and only then on a basically social level, not actively seeking referrals.

It's a good thing we did. For one thing, it gave Ned an opportunity to do a lot of reading and reflecting, and he dealt with a number of issues involving the human spirit and relationships. A few of his key relationships improved substantially, and he built a new perspective on life, which gave him greater peace of mind.

For another, Ned's conversations with a friend who had been successful in a different segment of retailing, were not only very calming, reassuring and full of positive reinforcement, but they also led to a referral on the West Coast. It seems a fellow there had built a profitable men's clothing chain, but needed another capable executive to help him grow it to the next stage. The situation was made to order for Ned, and he was hired as President.

He contacted me a year later to let me know that all aspects of his life were now quite satisfying and continuing to improve.

He's another among a long list of "Silver Lining" clients who say they would never wish their disability on themselves, but that a number of good things eventually resulted from it.

Pursuing the Opportunity Collision

Mary J was an exceptionally competent attorney with severe allergy problems. She had worked in a high-rise building in a major city, and while it wasn't a "sick building," its air conditioning system put out air that set off her allergies to the point where she couldn't work. She found that to be the case in most high-rises.

One of the few places in the country where she found relief was on a section of California's southern coast, where she could swim regularly, and where some of the office buildings were just one or two stories high, often with windows that opened to let in fresh ocean breezes. She decided to move there, and relocated to one of the more desirable coastal cities.

When I met her, she had already requested a settlement from the insuror that she considered sufficient to meet her financial needs while she established a practice in a new state. Part of her settlement was to have my services in helping her get established. We implemented a job search locally, with the proposition that she could work in a number of important behind-the-scenes functions for a law firm until she was admitted to practice law in California.

With her confident and creative personality, she remained open to any opportunities that might come her way, regardless of whether they fit her idea of the ideal position. With each passing week her physical condition improved in the coastal environment, and she was able to energetically pursue a number of options.

It was this combination of open perspective and enthusiastic implementation that led to an unexpected opportunity. One of the largest law firms in the town she had selected needed to hire an Administrator. But they had determined that this position would be unusual. Not only would the individual manage the business operations of the firm, but also serve as public spokesperson, helping to set and implement policy with respect to public and community relations, as well as coordinating the firm's efforts to attract new clients.

Mary had achievements in each of these areas with her previous firm, and the job was well suited to her personality. The multi-aspected nature of the job appealed to her, and she decided to accept the position, even though she would not be functioning as an attorney. There was an understanding that if she wanted to function as an attorney after she'd been in the job for a year, she could train someone else for her position, and make the move then.

Six months later she was still feeling good about the move, and feeling better than ever physically. By remaining open to *The Opportunity Collision,* she apparently found a position that was exceptionally well suited for her.

Rebounding From an Emotional Low

There will always be a special place in my heart for Don K. A young man in his late 20s, he was referred to me by an insuror after they got a report from a local agency in the midwest that Don was not motivated or cooperative, and was probably depressed, even though his disability was a physical one related to back pain.

I never met Don, but in our first conversation he expressed

what seemed to me to be a very sincere desire to find a good job, and he didn't feel the kinds of jobs he'd been looking at were challenging. He considered them dead-ends. I explained I might be able to help him get a better job if he had experience and achievements that would impress a potential employer, and asked him to tell me some of the good things he'd done, how he'd improved things for previous employers.

What I heard impressed me, so I asked him to fill out my information-surfacing forms, which he did quickly and returned them to me. Based on that information, I was able to construct an accurate resume highlighting many achievements which would qualify him to manage a retail operation, or some aspect of a business. I also created some letters Don could use as the first step in contacting potential employers, and in implementing the other action avenues as well.

These materials really boosted Don's morale, as he saw for the first time in writing just how much he had contributed, and how creative he'd been in coming up with good solutions to business problems in the past. We agreed on a simple action plan that he could implement quickly, and with each action step his enthusiasm grew.

It was only six weeks before he had an offer for what he considered an ideal position, managing the operations side of a local service business involved with commercial building maintenance and the repair of equipment.

Getting Past The Problem of Being Stuck in One Industry

In one form or another, Joe A from Virginia had been in car sales, or Finance and Insurance related to car sales, for most of the previous ten years before his disability, back and leg problems, which resulted from a car accident. Joe had recovered enough to start looking for another job, and approached his insuror to see if they could provide any assistance. That's when I was asked to work with him.

We created two resumes, one for sales or sales management, and the other for operations manager in a service, financial or "information" industry. We also developed letters that focused on the future and what Joe could do for an employer. We targeted away from automotive sales because, with a few exceptions, Joe felt the dealers in his area didn't have opportunities with a promising long-term future.

Joe used all four action avenues, and interviewed for a number of positions outside the auto industry. Because he had to write a lot of letters, he purchased a used computer and developed some skill in using it. But over a period of eight months, he wasn't able to get a single offer.

During that time he even approached car dealers he thought might provide long-term personal growth, but got no offers. Joe suspected that one bad relationship from his past might be the cause of his problems in the auto industry. Fortunately we never got the chance to find out.

That's because Joe had refused to let himself be limited to autos, and had come to think of himself as a sales-oriented manager who could function well in most industries. It was that mindset that opened an ideal opportunity for him. Two people he had met through friends owned an unusually successful computer store at a time when many were failing. They handled a lot of sophisticated problems for their customers, who relied on their special expertise.

They wanted to open a second store that would target non-sophisticated users, again offering some unusual services and advice to people in that market, as they did in their existing operation. But they had no time to manage it, and realized that the best person to manage it would be someone who had recently learned computers and could therefore relate to the average customer. They hadn't found that person, so they hadn't opened the second store.

They were discussing this missed opportunity in front of Joe and his friend when, without a moment's hesitation, Joe told them they had just found the ideal person, so they should now move ahead. Within two months he was managing their newly opened store. During that time he had learned much more about pc's, but when he didn't have an answer he knew it was just a phone call away.

It's unusual for people to call me a year after we've completed our work together, but Joe did. He wanted me to know that, despite all the bad news about retail computer stores, the one he managed was flourishing, and he'd hired two people. More important from his perspective, he'd now shown he could function well even in technically demanding businesses, so that whatever happened to computers, the credibility he had gained gave him greater job security than ever before.

Moving From Clerical to Management .....
With an Unexpected Employer

Linda P was an exceptionally competent New York City woman in her late 30s, but she'd been underemployed for the past five years, working in secretarial and clerical positions for a major broadcasting company, after taking time out to care for her children. Ten years earlier she had held a variety of highly responsible positions in a family construction firm that built many types of commercial structures.

I was asked to help her find a new position after she was sufficiently recovered from painful gastrointestinal problems that had caused her to go on disability. As we began to work together, it quickly became apparent that she really didn't want to go back to a secretarial position, yet she had lost her confidence for taking on the kinds of responsible jobs she had held in the past.

I've never had any success helping a person go after a job they weren't excited about, so that left us one option -- to go after a more responsible position. We worked first to restore her self-confidence. Filling out the information forms helped a lot. Discussions in which she had to admit she'd really done all those good things helped a lot more. And seeing the resumes and letters finished the job.

There were two resumes, one positioning her for facilities management, (you don't necessarily have to emphasize your most recent experience if it doesn't help), and the other for office management. Linda had to admit she was well qualified for both positions, and either one would be satisfying.

Over the next four months she implemented one of the most creative and well thought out job searches I've had the pleasure to work on, uncovering dozens of potential opportunities with architectural and construction firms, consulting firms, and many other types of companies. In the course of doing so, she got back to the broadcasting company as instructed, to make sure she'd have the right kind of enthusiastic references.

And the unexpected happened.

The new resumes combined with a few well-rehearsed CARE stories had the desired effect, but not with the employers for which they'd been intended. Instead, more than a few people at the broadcasting company now saw her in an entirely new light. For the first time they appreciated all the talents she'd had but never used while working there. And one of them referred her to the Facilities Manager.

Within two weeks Linda was working in a position three levels higher than the one she'd had when she was forced to go on disability. She was heavily involved in creating new sets for shows hosted by famous personalities, working closely with them, and loving it. At the same time she coordinated the refurbishing of offices owned by the company in many parts of midtown New York. The versatility demanded by this job equaled that of her previous position in the construction firm. She was where she felt she belonged, and she'd never been more productive.

It's rare that a person can move up so dramatically in the same company, especially after a disability. What happened? Well, as Linda pointed out six months later at lunch with her husband and me, her experience hadn't changed, but the way she looked at it and talked about it sure had. And when she started to believe in herself once again, it was easy to make believers out of other people.

12.
AND FINALLY MORE PEOPLE WHO'VE GOTTEN JOBS,
And Taught Me About .....

Reassessing Where You Fit at Age 56

Imagine this. You're 56 years old. You're significantly overweight. You've been out of work for two years on disability, diagnosed as severe depression, but you come back to the point where you're considered okay to return to work. When you go out after a job, you are totally unsuccessful, even though your resume shows that as a reporter you covered high level events and personalities in the nation's capital.

Likely as not, you wouldn't be feeling too confident or optimistic. That's how it was for Harry C when I met with him in Virginia. Fortunately, it turned out he was creating a lot of his own problems. He was limiting himself by thinking he could work only for one of the major networks. And by including on his resume the names of famous personalities and events, he was giving employers the impression he'd be happy only with a top position that had lots of visibility, even though that wasn't the case.

And he hadn't given careful thought to the many valuable things he could do for other types of news-related organizations with his years of experience. Once we identified them, Harry realized that, while news and broadcasting had changed dramatically since he last worked, there were still plenty of niches where he'd fit quite well, and where he could make important contributions.

We created letters that focused on these areas of future contributions, rather than a resume that focused on the past. Harry lost over 60 pounds. We worked on an interview approach that included a lot of CARE stories. His confidence and self-esteem took off on a vertical climb, and he started to open up opportunities in the less glamorous but highly challenging segments of the broadcast industry.

Within six months he had won what he considered the ideal job - a position as Executive Producer for a company that produced video news releases for major associations and other organizations. He had succeeded against what he had considered some pretty high odds - until he realized a lot of the odds were only in his own mind. He was now the proud possessor of a new and positive outlook on life.

Beating a Disability, a Reference Problem, and a Lousy Resume

Tyrone N had been a youth counselor in Washington DC, and a good one. When I met him, he had already beaten a physical disability associated with lower back pain, taking a little over a year to do it. But he wasn't successful in getting a new job, so the insuror asked me to help.

I soon learned that he had not only been an excellent counselor, but had also developed and put in place new methods, procedures, and programs that were very successful in practical working situations, and had been selected to receive special instruction at a national training academy, after which he had created even more innovative programs.

But none of this was on the resume. It came out only after discussions based on my information-surfacing forms. The resume we then put together gave a clear picture of a truly outstanding performer, and Tyrone began to get a lot of interviews for positions he wanted. But he wasn't getting any offers.

To our surprise, we learned he was getting a bad reference from a previous boss. Why? No good reason, really. Mainly it was a case of the boss feeling she was made to look bad by comparison to Tyrone's achievements, and was improperly labeling him "difficult to manage."

There are standard things you do in such instances. First, you try to avoid the reference, and you make sure the other references emphasize the opposite of what the bad reference says. If that doesn't work, you explain to employers that you had an honest disagreement with that person, and describe the situation from your vantage point, attempting to "defuse" it. If that doesn't work, you directly confront the bad reference, and ask them to stop. If that doesn't work, you need to make it clear you're being deprived of making a livelihood and will be forced to legal action.

In Tyrone's case, we only had to go the first two steps, avoiding the bad reference and making sure the others emphasized how easy he was to manage. Within weeks, he had an offer that combined counseling and management, which is what he wanted.

Making It In a Man's World -- Twice

Lillian W had risen through the ranks to hold a

responsible position in materials management, production scheduling and control, with a major food processor in the Pacific Northwest, the only woman ever to do so in that facility. But a lot of people resented her, even though she had a delightful personality. When I spoke with her by phone, she'd been out for more than a year with a physical disability, but there had also been an overlay of depression, due to some bad experiences on the job, compounded by marital and family problems that resulted in divorce.

Although I never met Lillian, I came to respect her as an especially resilient personality, who was capable of putting bad experiences behind her and getting on with life, choosing to take a positive perspective about the future.

There was no job for her with her previous employer, and she wasn't sure whether she wanted to go back into production, seek out a position in Accounting, where she'd taken many courses, or switch to sales and customer service, taking advantage of her pleasing personality and what reports had indicated were her good looks (confirmed some time later by a photo she sent me of Lillian holding her two-year-old daughter).

Our solution was the *Close Encounter With Stated Goals,* and I created resumes and letters for Lillian which positioned her for each of the three options. Despite the fact that she was hard-pressed financially and couldn't afford to live on her own, she was exceptionally diligent in implementing all four action avenues.

I don't think she could have done it without the computer-generated information on employer prospects I had provided, or without the help of her parents, who happened to be my age. Her mother served as her "search coordinator." She and I became "phone friends" over time.

Eventually Lillian uncovered opportunities in both Oregon and Washington. She accepted one that lasted just a few weeks. The employer had misrepresented some aspects of the job, and hadn't informed her about the active opposition the primarily female work force in that part of the plant would put up against any female boss.

After a number of months Lillian found the ideal job in Seattle. Once again, she had chosen production in the food industry, even though she also had an offer for an accounting position. This time, though, she had done her homework and knew she'd be working in an environment in which she'd be appreciated for her abilities.

She was right. The last I heard from her, she'd already gotten a promotion, was living on her own, happier on the job than she'd ever been, was enjoying her daughter, and had two handsome fellows proposing marriage.

Making an Unexpected Switch -- Geographically and Career-wise

I'll never forget Jack R, if only because my meeting with him involved the smoothest car trip I've ever had coming back from New England. It started at midnight after a snowstorm, and I don't believe I saw more than a dozen other cars on the 250 miles of newly cleared highways until I got into the Metropolitan New York City area.

I had met with Jack at his home in southeast New Hampshire, after the insuror had asked me to help him. Before he hurt his back, his most recent positions had been in inventory control and production scheduling for an electronics manufacturer. He had been working with an agency in New

Hampshire that helped him find a production job with a roofing company, but it hadn't lasted more than a few weeks.

Because I was traveling to Massachusetts anyway, I'd arranged to meet him almost as soon as he was referred, with no opportunity for him to complete my information-surfacing forms. So he provided me the information verbally over his kitchen table. I've learned not to be surprised by what I learn in such instances.

Given Jack's outgoing personality, I wasn't really surprised to learn that he also had some sales experience. Still in his early thirties, he had a nice blend of experience that covered sales, production, materials, and purchasing. I explained that this opened up many different kinds of opportunities, including that of general management for a small company.

Jack hadn't really thought much about his sales experience before, and really hadn't considered himself qualified to be a general manager, no matter how small the company. As we discussed the specifics of his achievements, however, he had to admit that he had experience in all the component parts of management, and probably was qualified after all.

We created two resumes and a number of letters that enabled him to pursue different types of positions, since he wasn't sure what he wanted. Our computer search for employer prospects included parts of New England and the Tampa/ Clearwater area in Florida, where he thought he might want to live if he decided to relocate.

One of the key things I taught Jack was to tell CARE stories that got across how he had initiated new procedures or made improvements in old ones to increase productivity, and how he had won new customers in sales.

His resumes and letters opened up opportunities in New England and Florida, and he used his CARE stories well to impress prospective employers. The most promising position was in Florida, where he became General Manager of a small electronic component manufacturer that couldn't afford both a sales manager and a production manager, so they got two for the price of one in Jack. Two years later Jack told me that the company had grown, and he was forced to admit he'd done a good job as General Manager.

Gaining New Direction from the *Close Encounter*

Seemingly by coincidence, I had two California clients at the same time who both chose new directions after a *Close Encounter With A Stated Goal*. Ronnie L thought he wanted to start a sales training business for route salesmen, using the techniques he had learned to become very productive in such a position over the years. His arm injury wouldn't keep him from doing it effectively, he reasoned, and a lot of companies with route salespeople had already expressed strong initial interest when he had approached them.

So I quickly put together a first draft for a brochure, created letters that would serve as initial contacts with prospects, and developed a step-by-step action plan that would have him contacting prospects within two weeks. When I didn't hear from him after three weeks, I called, suspecting something had happened.

It had. As soon as he got my materials, Ronnie realized he could be in business the following week, and it brought home to him some strong feelings that he really didn't want to do sales training anymore. He never would have realized it unless he got close enough to actually feel it, he said, but now he was sure that what he really wanted was ..... jewelry repair !! He'd always enjoyed it as a hobby, and now he planned to take a job with a local jeweler, perhaps opening up his own business at some point in the future.

It was pretty much the same kind of experience for Dorothy V. Until her stress disability, she had done an outstanding job for an investment banking firm, heading up their automated office operations and managing conferences and events they sponsored. She now felt she wanted to either sell some of the sophisticated equipment she used to purchase, or become active in public relations.

So I created two resumes for her, and some letters, and promised two more resumes for other directions she wanted to pursue, but asked for her feedback from the first two before starting the others. Well she loved the resumes, she told me, but they'd had an unintended effect.

As she read them, she began to realize it was likely she could actually win one of those jobs, and that made her face squarely her current priorities, values, and life goals. When she did, she knew she didn't want any part of the stress that went with the types of jobs she originally said she wanted. But she found that out only after "getting close" emotionally to the prospect of winning those jobs.

The option she chose was a new field at the time, fingernail painting. She intended to work first in the shop of another woman, and then she planned to open her own shop. It gave her an outlet for her creativity, and instead of stress, the daily working environment was one that she found to have a beneficial healing effect on her, physically and mentally.

I told her it was wise to follow her own inner instincts, but that if she tired of the fingernail painting, or wanted to try something more aggressive in the future, to be sure to get back to me. She thanked me, volunteering she never would have known what she really wanted if we hadn't gone through our process, and said she'd be sure to get back if and when things changed. She never got back.

Whenever there's a seeming coincidence, such as having Ronnie and Dorothy as clients at the same time, with almost identical results, I feel that life is trying to teach me something, and I look for the lesson to be learned.

Maybe the lesson here is that *Close Encounters* can sometimes lead to totally unexpected directions, and even when they appear to make little sense at first, if they feel right, they're worthwhile following through. There's usually a sound logical reason why we have impulses that seem to come out of nowhere, and the unexpected often turns out to be quite suitable.

13.
SOME PEOPLE WHO STARTED BUSINESSES

.....

That Seemed To Fit

It was about five years ago when the trend toward my clients choosing to go into business really accelerated. I learned early on that it didn't pay to assume a business wasn't feasible just because it was unusual. Almost always, when people approached an insuror and requested assistance in getting a business off the ground or buying into one, they had valid reasons for believing in the business. And they often had special talents or knowledge that gave them an edge.

But even in those few cases where they didn't, they had determination, and that's the single factor that impressed me the most. One way or another, all of these people were determined to get into a business. Some built that determination only after they realized they couldn't get a job they would like. Others had it from the start. Regardless, they persevered, often despite obstacles, until they were in a business.

And that business just seemed to fit them, even if it was one they hadn't thought about until after they had first considered other businesses. In retrospect, we'd wonder why it wasn't the first business they looked it, it would seem such a natural. I suppose going through the search was a method of forcing themselves to focus on what they really wanted. Score one for the *Close Encounters* approach.

Here are some stories about people who started or purchased businesses. Unfortunately, the nature of my relationships with clients is such that I'm there to assist them at a certain critical time, but normally we don't maintain contact after that. At least I know they started off on the right foot, with a sound plan, enough capital to last them until projected breakeven, and an analysis that indicated they had a reasonable chance to succeed.

The Ultimate Test of The Close Encounter Approach ?

As I've mentioned earlier, my basic approach with clients is to help them find something to get excited about, then provide them whatever they need to "get close" to it, so they can find out firsthand whether they still want it when they're "up close" to it. If the chosen option loses its appeal, that's considered progress, because we've eliminated a "phantom option" and can proceed to get close to the next one, and so on, until we find the one that's right. I call this approach *Close Encounter With Stated Goals.*

In most instances, after two or three "close encounters," we're able to find a suitable option. But not so with Dan V in the Pacific Northwest. His is an interesting case in many ways, not just because it required so many "close encounters," but because of the range of emotional reactions and belief systems he went through. In the beginning I had to do much more pushing than I'm accustomed to, but by the end, he was pulling me along with his enthusiasm.

Dan was a self-employed tree cutter in his late 30s who developed back and leg pain after an operation for herniated discs. He could no longer cut trees, but in theory at least there were other types of jobs he could perform. We concentrated initially on finding a job, but jobs are not plentiful in the part of the country where he lives. Almost all timber related jobs have disappeared, and the region is not densely populated. It would require an intense effort.

Yet it was difficult to get him to cooperate. He put very little information on my forms, other than to say that all he'd ever done was cut trees. Relying on my own knowledge of what it takes to run a business of that nature, I put together a resume for him that showed he had experience in sales, customer relations, bidding, operations, administration, project management, supervision, and quality standards. The resume positioned him as someone who could manage all or part of the operations of many different types of small businesses, since that appeared to be the option which held the most promise.

As I often do, I also created letters to show him how he could take the first step in communicating with people, using the four basic action avenues we had discussed. When I got no response, I figured something was wrong, so I called. I remember the conversation well, because I was traveling on business in Florida at the time. It was one of those knock-down, drag-out conversations with a lot of long pauses, a type I don't especially enjoy.

He just wouldn't believe he had those skills I'd highlighted, or that he could really manage some aspect of another person's business. I kept going back to the facts, asking him if he hadn't done this or that, and he had to admit that he had. But in his mind, that didn't mean he could do it for someone else in a different business.

The conversation was a standoff at best. My bottom line on it was that if he truly couldn't function outside tree cutting, and there were no jobs in tree cutting, we'd be foolish to take any actions at all. But I let him know I didn't share his beliefs and didn't agree with the limits he had placed on himself.

I received this referral in March, and it took me until May to convince him he could in good faith present himself as someone capable of managing a business, or even part of it. And the only reason I could achieve that was because the insuror was good enough to make a special provision to reimburse him for travel and childcare expenses while he worked free-of-charge if necessary for two months while he learned someone's business. We had to offer that in order to take away his many objections - shamed him into it, in a sense.

Taking action has a way of putting things in proper perspective. As he began to make direct personal contacts with business owners and managers, he gradually developed greater appreciation for his array of talents and the variety of business settings in which they could be profitably applied. He could actually see himself contributing in auto parts, highway construction, retail clothing, a deli / food store, an electronics distributor, sporting goods store, and others he got close to.

Problem was, even with his wife working, money was tight. Most jobs would leave him financially worse off than staying on benefit, the classic financial disincentive. Relocation was out of the question for a number of reasons. His small town offered few opportunities, the nearest sizable town was over 40 miles away, and a major city was twice that distance.

Despite these obstacles, we had now developed some momentum. The distance you cover when you go from believing you have nothing to offer, to believing you have something to offer but no place to sell it, is infinite.

We discussed the practical realities of job search and concluded he might be better off if he could offer to purchase all or part of a business, instead of just trying for a job. I got back to the insuror and they agreed that, if we could find a suitable business I evaluated as feasible, they'd be positively disposed to consider a settlement.

Which was good news, except that his circumstances and policy terms indicated only a relatively small settlement, not enough to acquire most businesses. I wasn't able to provide him anything but a broad range as guidance, but suggested he proceed nevertheless, and he did. The businesses he looked at included a fish farm, trailer park, espresso bars, delis, and a variety of retail and wholesale businesses.

His frustration grew as businesses either didn't fit him emotionally, in the sense that he couldn't relate to them, or more often the case, he simply couldn't afford them. In that part of the country, successful businesses sold at higher multiples than the norm. He'd now had well over a dozen "close encounters," and was beginning to doubt whether he'd ever find anything he could enjoy that would also meet his financial goals.

So far we'd struck out on jobs, and on buying into existing businesses, so I suggested he look into starting a business another client in that part of the country had operated, the mobile mill business, where you truck a sawmill to a site and turn logs into lumber for customers, or sell the wood to someone else. I provided written details of how the business worked, the cost structure, markets, and cost of entry, which was relatively low. We also discussed how he could operate it differently from the other fellow, because they were in quite different circumstances.

Enthusiasm took hold, and this once sullen client turned into an upbeat, optimistic, confident person, who thoroughly researched the business and lined up customers who would definitely buy in quantities and at prices that would virtually guarantee the desired profit levels.

He had to nail down only one thing - a dependable source of supply of fallen trees - and he knew from past experience that the Forest Service sold more than enough on a regular basis, at exceptionally low prices.

Or at least he thought he knew. Anything can be taken to an extreme. The environmental laws are basically necessary, and there for a good reason, but in this case they'd been taken to an extreme. The amount of paperwork the Forest Service is required to fill out for environmental purposes is now so great that they refuse to sell access to fallen trees unless a large contract is involved. Otherwise, it just doesn't pay, and they'd prefer to let the wood rot on the ground.

Scratch the mobile mill business. Who could have guessed - plenty of willing customers, but no source of supply!

At this point I had frankly run out of ideas. But my client had transformed from the reluctant job seeker to the indefatigable pursuer of business opportunities. Once again, my theory comes into play, that when people expend a great deal of energy and emotion pursuing something, and almost make it happen but it doesn't work out, then inevitably something else will pop up very quickly that is just as appealing.

Theory or no, in this case it happened. Three women, friends of the client's wife, had built a part-time business over the past three years, silk screening T-shirts, children's items, and corporate gifts and clothing, to the point where it made a profit of about $10,000. But it was taking over their lives, requiring all their spare time, and they wanted to sell it - for about the amount of money it made in a year, which was just a little more than the equipment cost!

My client was very active in Little League and other children's sports, and had been an athlete in school as well as in a semi-pro league. In years past a relative with a sporting goods store had been successful in selling uniforms to athletic teams, traveling throughout the region selling to schools and municipalities. The current owner of the sporting goods store didn't go after that business, and didn't want to. My client figured he could travel the region, take advantage of his many sports-related contacts, and supplement the existing silk screen business with uniform sales.

The more he researched it, the better it looked. Coaches he knew gave him virtual commitments. The sporting goods store was happy to purchase the uniforms for him from the best supplier, for a small percentage of the profits. (That supplier sold only to sporting goods stores.) Taverns and softball teams said they'd buy. Golf courses were interested. And businesses liked the idea of the personal attention and speed of delivery he offered. The three women would make sure he kept all existing accounts.

Based on his input and some information I asked him to gather, I put together a simple plan and analysis with income projections and startup costs. It showed he had a reasonable chance to reach his financial goals in this business he was so excited about, if a settlement could provide enough for startup costs and a supplement to his first six months' earnings. The analysis indicated an absolute minimum amount required for feasibility, another amount that I considered more adequate, and another larger amount that the client said he would like.

The insuror came back with an offer for the amount I considered adequate, the client was obviously pleased and outspokenly appreciative for the assistance he'd gotten, and as for me - I thanked my Guardian Angel !!! Maybe that's giving the angel too much credit, but we had help from somewhere on this one.

The Rehab Coordinator showed extreme patience, and the insuror was willing to go the extra mile when it meant go or no-go. It was a happy ending all around, but I'll be honest, I wouldn't wish that one on myself again. It's hard to believe the whole thing lasted less than six months. It seemed like years. And more close encounters than even a space alien would welcome.

Would You Believe A Family Reunion Yearbook Publishing Company?

Many times during the past few years, after listening to one of my rehab customers describe the business being planned by an insured, I was convinced the business had little or no chance of success, and figured I'd do the person a good turn by persuading them to look at other options. I've learned not to jump to quick conclusions anymore.

Why? Well, would you believe a family reunion yearbook publishing company, proposed by a fellow who had been a Ranch Manager? I figured it was some guy putting together a few pages for friends, who mistakenly thought he could make a business out of it. Rick B had other ideas.

How was I to know that just 30 miles from his home in rural Arkansas there was a now-famous entertainment city, and a nearby center that hosted hundreds of family reunions every year, each with hundreds of participants and 150 decision makers who were happy to spend $30 each for a book?

And who would suspect that it only costs a fraction of that amount per book before printing, and this you collect up front? And that the "Ancestral Fair," a kind of convention for these reunion people, had over 800 people register? And that you can get to these people with no expensive advertising? And that Rick was skilled enough in computer operation to turn out a truly superior competitive book?

As it turns out, financial projections for the first 24

months were so impressive, Rick would be earning more in this business than he did on his job, if he did just 30% of what we expected he could do. Sure, he had some pain and some limited mobility, but not so much that he couldn't operate this business. I believe he would have found a way to operate it regardless of any physical limitations in his way. It was too good a business not to.

And Then There Was Bill H, Who Wanted to Build and Repair Bamboo Fishing Rods.

Nice dream, I thought, Bill's idea of semi-retirement. Really didn't look forward to bursting his bubble. Turns out I needn't have worried. How was I to know there was a catalog that sold out in 16 weeks its entire stock of bamboo fishing poles, and that they would cut a deal with Bill where they would do all the marketing and advertising and give him a percentage of the profit that would nearly equal his previous income if he made just half the poles he was capable of making?

And how was I to know Bill was smart enough to check out potential competition, all three of them in the U.S., and learn that they were all doing very nicely, thank you, and that they were increasing their prices as they got better known? And that people would spend more on those poles than I would on a bicycle? And that the raw materials might be purchased for $15? I managed to raise a number of good questions, but he went and got the answers. I understand he settled, and went into this unusual but viable business.

Here's One of My Favorites ..... Horse Art.

Betty S in California is a charming woman with lupus. Formerly a graphic arts supervisor, she also did beautiful artwork, but only about horses, and wondered if she could make a business of it. Initial discussions indicated she might have a chance marketing clothing and other items to the horse show market, so I called in a woman to work with me who knows horses and clothing.

That was two years ago. From a standing start, and working only as long and hard as her lupus would allow, Betty built a network of suppliers, became knowledgeable about pricing, gained some publicity, enjoyed a lot of referral work, and stands a good chance of earning a significant profit within the next two years.

That's a long time by some standards, but when you compare it to the alternative, sitting around doing nothing, it's not so bad. My involvement here was minimal ... a simple plan of action, a lot of encouragement, identifying the right sub-consultant, coordinating her input, and providing a few good ideas here and there.

Like most successful clients, she needed only a few months of concentrated effort, and then she was off on her own, with just an occasional call. She's one of dozens of people around the country who consider me a good friend, whom I never get to meet face-to-face. Thankfully, the phone does a good job of conveying the spirit, and that counts for more than faces.

Coffee and Sandwiches, Anyone?

Does history repeat itself? In the case of Mike Z, after about 5 years, it did. When Mike became a client, it had been about that long since I helped another client sort through his options and decide on investing in a luncheonette in Massachusetts.

The Rehabilitation Coordinator who referred Mike to me was concerned about him. He was in his early 30s, also lived in Massachusetts, and wanted to settle his claim in order to get the cash he'd need to invest in a franchise in the child safety business. She asked me to determine whether the business was a viable one for him.

Mike was a hard working and highly motivated fellow, with a pleasant personality. His previous job had been that of route salesperson for a bakery company, and the disability was disc herniation, which prevented him from lifting the loads his job required. He had already made a small investment in a vacuum cleaner franchise, but it had failed, principally because he wasn't effective in that type of sales.

We were able to define his many strengths, and compare them to the opportunities he was seeking. The child safety franchise, for example, required intense conceptual selling over a long period, and he simply wasn't cut out for that type of sales. Further analysis showed that, even if he were, he'd have to travel so far to make his sales presentations, it wouldn't be a viable business.

Over the next two months we analyzed a variety of franchises and businesses for sale, and he gradually became knowledgeable about the relative price/earnings multiples being paid for businesses in his area, the essential questions he had to have answers for before evaluating a business properly, and the kinds of future events that might affect a business's viability. Concentrating on businesses that did not require a "hard sell," we eventually settled on sandwich shops and vending routes as possibilities.

While investigating a franchise that looked promising, he learned of a sandwich/coffee shop in his hometown that was located in a prime office building. When a business of that nature is available, it can be a good solution for someone who wants to "buy a job" by buying a business. It should have a history of stable earnings, or if not, a positive recent trend, and the purchaser needs to make sure there are no future developments such as construction or the closing of a nearby factory, that might significantly reduce revenues.

Initial figures provided by the current owner left a lot of questions unanswered, so I directed my client to get those answers, check for possible rent increases or major tenants leaving the building, then review the entire deal with a local accountant and lawyer.

If he did decide to move ahead, I suggested a certain method of purchase, with which his accountant agreed. What at first appeared to be an asking price of 2.5x earnings, on closer examination was less than 1.5x earnings, with terms, which his accountant and lawyer agreed was a good deal for him.

The business is well-suited for him in many ways. His settlement plus some money a relative put in, covers the cost of the business. The current owner, who has a stake in his success because of future payments, helped him get established.

Thanks to one very caring Rehab Coordinator who took the initiative to make sure he'd be investing in a business with a good chance of succeeding, Mike bought a stable business with a reasonably bright future, instead of losing money by investing in a business that he had little chance of making successful.

Getting An Architectural Consulting Business Off the Ground

Joe U is an architect in the Los Angeles Area, a talented man in his 30s who had played a key role on major projects for a leading international firm. The disability involved extreme vertigo, dizzy spells, ringing in the ears, facial twitches and, most significant from a vocational perspective, very low levels of energy and stamina.

He thought he could plan for a slow, gradual, long-term return to work as a consultant to other architects, while perhaps doing some local work as an architect, working out of his home, contracting out the portions he couldn't handle physically.

Problem was, Joe needed training on some things he used to have others do for him, plus computer hardware, software, and money to operate a vehicle. That came to a total somewhat less than $20,000. He had done his homework on calculating expenses, but he hadn't really thought through how he would win business. His "plan" that he submitted to the insuror was a plan for how he would spend that money to acquire new talents, but said nothing about how, when, and with whom he expected to win assignments.

Probably due in large measure to his disability, he had little patience for discussing the subject, and seemed both annoyed and disheartened that he couldn't just be given the money without a plan.

A number of discussions ensued, and there were many delays. In one discussion with the Coordinator, I voiced my opinion that chances for making real progress here were remote. He understood the problem, urged me to continue my dialogue with the client, and made direct contacts himself to lend encouragement and provide motivation.

Somewhere in that process, we broke through. We don't know who said what, or if anything that was said really mattered, but after a couple of months, Joe's attitude changed.

In our discussions we began to make real headway on identifying his markets, his special advantages, his "selling proposition," the special benefits he would bring to clients, and the methods he would use to win new business. Not only did he put together a simple, complete plan, he also willingly revised it three times to incorporate new ideas or to correct assumptions not supported by the facts.

And a funny thing happened. He began to feel a lot more energy, became less argumentative, less annoyed, more positive, and then *extremely appreciative* for the input of the Coordinator and me. His final plan was for five years, very realistic, and very well thought out. The Coordinator went to bat for him, got him the money he requested, and he moved quickly to implement.

But not before he volunteered that he knew he'd been tough to deal with, until he recognized that two people who really didn't know him that well were going out of their way to do what they could to help him become successful. That thought turned him around, he said, and gave him real confidence that he could not only reach his goals, but enjoy the energies that come with giving and receiving while getting there. The Coordinator's unflagging support for Joe made that happen.

As so often happens in these cases, the unexpected occurred. While starting his training and arranging other things to get his business started, Joe won a contract on a substantial project, something he hadn't expected for about two years. The result? He builds momentum, and the insuror enjoys a sizable offset far sooner than anticipated. Not bad for a situation I once thought was going nowhere.

A Little Goes A Long Way!

The point was made earlier that just a little input from someone else can often make a big difference in someone else's life. It seems that feeling good about yourself, having a resume that gets your best strengths across, getting a few new ideas, and just knowing there's someone out there who cares about you, can have a dramatic effect on people's effectiveness, whether they are top executives or just a step beyond entry level. Makes you realize the truth of Leo Buscaglia's words in *Born for Love,* which I referred to earlier, and how much they apply to our daily work, whatever it is .....

"The majority of us lead quiet, unheralded lives as we pass through this world. There will most likely be no ticker-tape parades for us, no monuments created in our honor. But that does not lessen our possible impact, for there are scores of people waiting for someone like us to come along; people who will appreciate our compassion, our encouragement, who will need our unique talents ... someone who will live a happier life merely because we took the time to share what we had to give. ... Too often we underestimate the power of a touch, a smile, a kind word, a listening ear, an honest compliment, or the smallest act of caring, all of which have the potential to turn a life around. It's overwhelming to consider the continuous opportunities there are to make our love felt."

There have been any number of times when people gave me credit for doing a lot more than I really did. One striking example was Lillian C, a woman in Florida with severe allergies, who had accomplished a lot in Loss Control and Safety Training. When I first spoke with her, she was attempting to build a medical transcription business she had started from home.

We had two good conversations, surfacing lots of ideas that were well suited to her situation, and over the phone I gave her some words to use in flyers and letters. Our third conversation started with her opening comment, "Well, you don't know what a torrent of creativity you've unleashed. Your ideas have stimulated my imagination, and I'm going great guns."

Indeed she was. She was expanding her operation to another city. She had called dozens of doctors, found effective new ways to get business, started operating in a more productive mode, recruited new word processors, established another business that wouldn't take much of her time, and created some flyers. She's one of the relatively few clients who stay in touch, and her business continues to prosper two years later.

And To Your List of Businesses You Never Knew About, Add.....

The high-priced dress business. Very high-priced!!! Tom R in Mississippi, in his 50s, would definitely not impress you as a retail sales hotshot. He had a manufacturing background. When I learned he wanted to go into business in Atlanta with his sister, selling dresses in a retail shop, I was skeptical to put it mildly.

I was asked to check it out, to determine if it was realistic for him, or whether he'd be better off in another line of work, which I was sure he would be. As mentioned earlier, I'm convinced. There is *always* a good reason why, when people want to go into an unusual business.

Seems his sister had started out selling dresses to country-western singing stars and beauty contestants, where they spend BIG money for dresses. She had moved to a major city in the South many years ago, and opened a shop where she now has a loyal clientele to whom she sells dresses ..... starting at $6000!!! (They stop at about $30,000.)

Well, seems the sister knew there is a strong pent-up demand in that city for European designer dresses in a more "modest" price range ... $400 to $2500! The plan was for her to finance the new shop, sending a lot of browsers from her shop to his, referring daughters of the wealthy women she serves, and providing all the initial inventory.

It's wonderful, the things you can find out with a few good questions. People never cease to amaze me with these unusual businesses, and they continue to educate me!! In this case, Tom knew the risks, and if ever a startup retail business had all the key leverage factors going for it, and a strong financial backing as well, this was it.

Of course it can fail. Any business can. But any prudent business person would love to have a startup with the realistic chance for success this one had. Eventually he chose another, more conventional option, but working on this one built momentum for him. It was "something to get excited about," and was a catalyst for his getting back into action.

As Time Goes By

Most of us have had at least one instance in their lives where we work very hard on something, think we're making tremendous progress, and look forward to successfully reaching our goal ..... but it doesn't happen. About two years ago a referral came my way that would have to be considered unusual by almost any measure.

Bob F from Cleveland was in his early forties, had been in the music promotion business, and had more physical problems in the previous four years than you'd want to handle in a lifetime. These included, but were not limited to, malignant lymphoma, pneumonia, upper and lower respiratory infections, kidney stones, hernias, bone cysts in one leg, a popped knee joint, chronic back pain and sciatica, and peritonitis.

Apparently at one point he was even considered dead for some minutes after an operation, but he made one of those miracle recoveries. In fact, Bob had come back to the point where, if you met him, you wouldn't know there was anything wrong with him. Not only that, but he also had a dynamic personality and a husky build, so you'd think he was the picture of good health, strong and energetic.

But he still had some operations ahead of him when he was

referred to me, so the Rehab Coordinator expected only some "advance planning" to help him focus on new options, with no real progress expected until the following fall at the earliest. After reading the file, I agreed. But we hadn't counted on the unusual degree of enthusiasm this fellow possessed. After just one phone call, he got excited and wanted me to come out to Cleveland and visit with him, which I was happy to do.

In that meeting, it turned out that the one thing he wanted to do more than anything else in the world was to join his long-time friend in the purchase of a radio station. His friend knew the business well, and their combined talents would make them an ideal management team.

So over the next few months we put together a sound plan (no pun intended), the excitement and energy continued to build, and it appeared that by the middle of the summer we'd have one very happy client reaching a settlement so that he could go into the business he loved, months ahead of the time when we were expecting to get started.

Problem was, when he got right up to it, he decided not to go ahead. Part of it was the risk, but there were other factors as well. So we dropped it, wished him well, and the insuror reassured him we knew he had been acting in good faith all along, and that this was a life decision which was his alone to make. For another month I stayed in touch to provide some guidance as he explored other alternatives.

I can't really say I was surprised when, six months later, he called to tell me he had three unusual opportunities offered to him, and felt strongly that he would want to take one of them.

The first was a restaurant that came as close to being a "sure thing" as a restaurant can. After 40 years a woman had shut it down because she couldn't find anyone she felt would love the business the way she did, and operate it accordingly. Until she met Bob and his proposed partner. They researched it and found that businesspeople in the area would almost immediately start begging them to reopen it. The second deal? A radio station, of course ... the ideal station. The third? A chance to buy into a well managed beauty salon.

A few weeks later he settled under terms essentially the same as those offered months earlier, but with a sense of calm and confidence replacing the earlier anxieties. There's a time for everything, he told me, and now was the time for him to settle and get on with his life, not last year and not next year. People seem to know when the time is right, and it isn't always according to our schedule.

Oh yes. He eventually invested in the beauty salon business, and the last I heard, he and his partner had expanded to two cities, employees were happier and more productive than ever because Bob is such a good person to work for, profits were up, and they had plans for expansion to several more cities over the next five years.

"A Man's Gotta Do What He's Gotta Do" ......
Even When It Appears To Have Very Limited Potential.

Harold B in Pennsylvania, who had suffered head trauma four years earlier while working in supermarket operations, was determined to get into the business of trading and selling used paperback mystery novels and a few other selected categories, from the Fifties and Sixties. He had reported about $300 profit from his first three months of operations, and the question put to me by the Rehabilitation Coordinator was, "Does this business have any potential?".

This was a "2-phone-call assignment," a type that I like

because we can often accomplish a lot in a very brief time. In my first call I learned that the business does have potential, but very little. I also learned that Harold was determined to do this business and none other. He had no interest in even discussing other options, and was quite satisifed with limited profits in the future.

When I got back to the Rehab Coordinator, we agreed that there are many positives to such a situation. Here we have a motivated claimant, pleased with his progress, and reaping a lot of psychological benefits from the activity. The obvious route is to offer support, to help him build the business as large as he can. Advances in sound, electrical and other technologies may or may not in the future enable him to advance beyond his current level of recovery. In the meantime, being active this way can only help, and he may raise his sights as time goes by.

I got back to Harold to provide advice on half a dozen ways he might build his list of customers. (In that business, revenues are directly related to the size of the customer list.) Over time those steps may help him build to a level where profit would be $350 to $400 per month. That's good enough for a first step. The offset helps the insuror a little. And momentum builds. You never know where it might lead. After doing what he's "gotta do," he may even want to try something else.

Some More Interesting Businesses People Have Gone Into Children's Fitness

Ron R in Florida, previously a commodities broker, decided to settle his claim so that he and his wife could start a business that had three separate parts to it. The biggest is children's fitness and gymnastics, a new business for them, though they researched it thoroughly. The second part is planning and directing parties for children, either at their homes or at the fitness center. Ron's wife has been in that business for two years, conducting the parties at the children's homes.

The third part of the business was manufacturing bounce houses, those air-filled houses the kids jump around in. As part of her party business, Ron's wife rented out a bounce house that she had purchased, and had little trouble keeping it fully rented out on weekends. Ron researched what would be required to make them, in order to sell them to others around the country who could rent them out as his wife did, and analysis showed it to be a viable proposition.

Espresso Carts

A client in the Seattle area, Jim N, previously worked in airline ramp operations. He originally wanted some help in setting up an interpreter business. But he soon realized he really didn't want to be in that business, and came back to the insuror instead with a plan to go into the espresso cart business.

It seems that espresso cart owners are on every street corner in Seattle, sometimes three or four thick, yet according to the input Jim got directly from them, they were all making a lot of money, as much as $10,000 per month, some claimed, and the required investment for a cart and coffee inventory is only about $15,000, substantially less than many businesses which don't earn a third of that reported income.

I checked with one of my insurance company customers in Seattle, and she verified that they were not only on the corners, but at gas stations, various stretches of highway, and in front of stores, with all of them seemingly doing a brisk business. She did not know why they were so popular in Seattle and hadn't caught on like that elsewhere. The client didn't know either, but intended to relocate to a Colorado resort town where they hadn't caught on yet.

I advised that he check first to see if town authorities would let him operate there, and whether he'd run into opposition from established businesses, then wished him luck. He knew it was a risk and wanted to take it.

Experience tells us that no business that simple will remain as profitable as reported for any extended period of time (the woman who runs one here in my town told me she doesn't make anywhere near the kind of money they do in

Seattle). But it's also true that if you're one of the first people in a good market with a service or product that catches on, you can make a lot of money quickly and get out of the business after a few years. Here's hoping that happens for Jim.

A Feed Store in the 1990s ?

A feed store in rural West Virginia? A growth business in the 1890s maybe, but in the 1990s? Most people would probably conclude that today it's sure to be a slow-growth or no-growth proposition. Not necessarily so, at least for Frank T, formerly a mining construction foreman, whose disability was a back problem, and who provides fresh custom feeds.

Frank wanted to settle to expand what had been his wife's business, which had tripled in two years. Seems the custom nature of the feeds and the fact that they are fresh, are very important factors for his customers. The fact that they'll deliver when competitors won't, is also a valuable plus. The core of customers they built provided the basis for a well-timed expansion in lawn and garden items. At last contact, their growth rate was proceeding smoothly.

Aptitude Testing and College Selection

Another promising business, for a client in Maryland who didn't need a settlement, was a combination of aptitude testing, college selection, and financial aid services for kids in high school and their parents.

Stan C, a former guidance counselor, was highly respected by parents and kids alike because his service is so highly personalized, and he maintained that this was the key difference between him and others in the field. He implemented what appeared to be a productive sales and marketing effort, for a large market that needs what he has to offer. Seems there's a business to fit every background.

Are We Limited Only By our Imagination?

It seems there is no end to the types of businesses people first think of, and then make a reality, based on their personal interests and talents. Yes, the disability will often limit the type of business they can run, or affect the way they have to operate, but just as often the disability itself will be the catalyst that leads them to the business in the first place.

At any rate, it seems not to limit their creativity or determination, and the businesses my clients enter in the future will likely be just as varied as those started in the past .....

catering ... convenience stores ... lobster hauling ... printing brokerage ... arranging meetings and conventions ... building custom furniture ... massage therapy ... selling automobile brakes ... sharpening saw blades ... training insurance salespeople ... investing in rental properties ...

tree pruning and cutting ... residential cleaning ... raising birds ... running a restaurant/bar ... a heating/ventilating/air conditioning contractor ... short-hauling stones with a tri-axle dump truck ... restaurant interior refurbishing ... liquor stores ... gas stations ... computer consulting

manufacturing false teeth ... a wireless subscription TV station ... making fudge and cookies ... operating a cabaret in a resort town ... shipping and transportation claims consulting ...

boarding homes for senior citizens ... repairing and making golf clubs ... management consulting ... child care centers ... filing medical claims ...

The possibilities appear to be as varied as people's natural talents and interests.

I keep having to remind myself that these businesses were all started by people who ..... experienced a disability significant enough so that they could no longer work in their chosen field ... got past the discouragement and often the pain ... turned a seemingly unfortunate event into a catalyst for something positive ... rebuilt their confidence and self-esteem ... mustered enough energy to visualize and plan a business they hadn't been in before ... then found the courage to move ahead and take actions that turned their ideas into reality.

Can you blame me for sometimes thinking I'm dealing with an exceptional group of human beings? Maybe they're just like everyone else, but the special difficulties they faced managed to bring out the best in them, and maybe that would happen with most of us. I'd like to think so. Regardless, it sure is inspirational to be around them, and I'm grateful for the chance to work with them.

14.
SO IS THERE ANYTHING IN ALL OF THIS
That Can Help You?

Stories about other people's success are not always a source of positive reinforcement. Sometimes they can increase a person's anxieties or depression by highlighting the gap between their own difficult situation and the enjoyable life experiences others have attained.

For any readers who might share some of that reaction, I can only point out that life is a very different experience for each of us. Comparing our progress or lack of it to others is usually an exercise in futility, particularly when it causes us anxiety.

The people I've observed who seem most content are those ... who don't look to others for approval ... who are quick to tell you that they are not on earth to meet anyone else's expectations ... who adopt the attitude that they are responsible for making the best out of any life situation they find themselves in ... and who are willing to take whatever actions are necessary to reach their goals.

I'm not saying I'd be able to do that, or that you necessarily should. All I can do is point to those who, in my experience, have achieved a measure of happiness despite a disability, and describe the characteristics they seem to share.

On the positive side, if there was one story in here that

you could relate to, or that helped you visualize yourself achieving something that maybe you'd thought you weren't capable of, then the effort of reading this was worth the while. If it helped you develop a perspective that gives you more peace of mind, even if you take no action to change anything, it was worth the while.

Over the years a lot of people have expressed relief just to learn that they are not the only ones having negative reactions to their situation. Or they were pleased just to have someone to share their fears and concerns with, and to know they could start to take action to get past them. Sometimes they expressed appreciation for being yanked a little closer to the world of action, jobs, and businesses, away from the isolation they'd gradually become accustomed to.

At times they found a particular framework of ideas, a certain way of looking at things, that gave them a more positive and hopeful perspective. And occasionally, they said they needed to travel through certain ideas and explorations just to attain peace of mind with their decision not to take any actions to change their personal circumstances.

The thoughts and stories here were presented with the hope that some of you might have similar positive reactions. If some of you have, then regardless of whether I ever learn about your reaction, you've presented me with a wonderful gift, and writing this was well worth the while.

15.
I'M STILL LEARNING ..... CAN YOU HELP ME?

Perhaps you've got a story to tell that others would find inspiring. It could be about yourself or someone you know. Maybe you've got a way of looking at things that helped you either get back into action, or made you feel a lot better about yourself and the world. A new idea might have occurred to you, or a new concept for an organization, a particular plan of action, or something you'd like to write.

I suppose I shouldn't be so loud in proclaiming that I've never had an original idea, but it's true. Many of the ideas I've shared have helped a lot of people, but not one of them was mine. The lives and thoughts of others are the raw material that I process and offer up as potentially helpful.

If they happen to hit the right person at the right time, some good has been done. So if you'd care to share something with others, please send it along, together with a note saying it's okay to mention it in discussions with others, or publish it in another book, or in a newsletter, and indicating whether it's okay to use your name, and whether you'd like others to get in touch with you.

Feedback will also be appreciated. If it's negative, I'll read it and then do my best to forget or suppress it right away. If it's positive, neutral, or contains "constructive criticism," it's a gift and I know I'll benefit by it, so thanks in advance.

(The next 11 pages are a reprint of instructions for filling out a worksheet.)

So You Want to Own a Business

Some Thoughts on Putting Together a Plan
Before You Start or Purchase a Business

It has been said by many entrepreneurs, that if they had foreseen at the outset all the problems they would encounter, they would never have started the business in the first place. Yet, looking back, they were glad they did. So you might ask yourself, why bother with a plan at all? In fact, unless your business is very complex or will require a number of investors, it's probably wise to stay away from a complicated business plan.

On the other hand, there are a few good solid reasons why you may want to have a simple plan. First, you'll have something to measure your progress by. If you are doing better or worse than expected, the plan may make it easier to find out why, so you can change things if necessary, or do more of the right things.

Second, it helps to know just how long you'll have to be putting money into a business before you start taking it out, so if your plan can tell you that ahead of time, you won't have any surprises. Surprises can be very painful in the area of cash flow.

Third, a plan forces you to start envisioning step-by-step how your business will proceed, so it begins to take on an emotional reality for you, and your feelings can tell you ahead of time whether a business is really for you. At the same time, it can help reveal any flaws in the way you propose to do business, and perhaps uncover a risk or two you hadn't thought of. Risks and flaws that are identified early can be corrected early, before much damage is done, improving your chances for success.

Answering the Basic Questions

A plan can be very simple, yet very effective, if it provides the answers to just a few basic questions. They are listed on the worksheet that accompanies these pages. Essentially, if you've got good answers to these questions, then you've got a good plan.

Please try to fill out the worksheet to the best of your ability, but don't be concerned if you don't have an answer or simply haven't given it much thought. This is just a starting point, and it gives us a clear indication of those areas where we may need to do some research or make some calculations. Here are some thoughts that may help stimulate your thinking as you answer each of the questions.

1. What Is the Nature of the Business?

Your answer may be obvious, but it is surprising to find how often people haven't thought this through. Sometimes the proposed business is a combination of two or three different businesses, and there has been no determination made with respect to how large a percentage each business will represent.

For example, a man intending to publish family reunion yearbooks also wanted to start a printing business, and a pennysaver publication, where he would be soliciting advertising. The three businesses are quite distinct, and in that case, it helped to figure out which would be the primary business, and when each one could realistically be started up.

In another case, a person wanted to go into the business of making and repairing golf clubs, but hadn't given much thought to what percentage of the business would be in repair work. This was important, because the profit ratios between building and repairing clubs were quite different.

So if your business can be explained simply in a sentence or so, please do so. If it involves more than one kind of activity, make sure you include them all. If you know what percentage you expect a particular segment of the business to be, put it down, but if you don't, you can simply mark, "Don't know."

2. Is There Really a Market Out There?

Sometimes the answer is obviously yes, especially if you are buying a business, or if others are already doing it and they are prosperous. At other times, people want to start up a business where they are not sure if there is really much demand out there. The easiest and fastest way to find out, is to go directly to the kind of people you would expect to be customers, and talk with them.

A man who wanted to rebuild bamboo fishing poles made one quick call to the publisher of a catalog that carried fishing poles, and found that there was indeed a market for what he intended to make, and when such poles were included in catalogs in the past, they sold out in a matter of weeks.

On the other hand, a woman who wanted to go into the decorative basket business found that, for the types of baskets she would want to produce, and the prices she would have to charge, there simply wasn't a market. Firsthand research of that nature can often give you immediate answers as to whether or not you really have a market out there.

3. How Big Is the Market?

It helps to know how big the market is, because then it's easier to figure out what share of the market you would have to get in order to reach your goals. A man in the Pittsburgh area researched the tree removal and trimming business and found that all six people in his area had 10 to 16 week backlogs.

Another man investigating the same business in the Philadelphia area found that two large companies dominated the business in his region, that smaller operators didn't have enough business, and a number of them had given up on the business in the last few years. In both cases, the market itself was plenty big enough, but getting into that market was another question.

If you have no idea of the size of your market, you might want to visit the business reference section of a local library, and look up statistics on Standard Metropolitan Statistical Areas, or contact an industry association, which you might find in *Encyclopedia of Associations*, or using a Dun & Bradstreet directory, you might be able to quickly tally up the revenues of others in the business in your area.

Sometimes franchise information is helpful, and sometimes visiting with prospective customers can give you a good idea of how much they would purchase, and how large your potential market might be. Sometimes calling on people in a similar business, but in another region of the country, can be helpful. If people don't feel you'll be a competitor, they can be forthcoming with a lot of valuable information.

4. How Do You Expect to Get Enough Sales In Order to Make the Business Feasible?

In many cases, a person's past experience or current activity is a good indicator that he or she will be able to generate sufficient sales. Often a person has a special advantage, such as a real estate person investing in rental properties, who gets a lead on the best buys, and also has connections with builders to get repairs made quickly and cheaply.

Sometimes a person has both a sales personality and lots of sales achievements, which indicate they would likely be successful. In other cases, the location is a reliable indicator of sales. This is especially true in retail businesses like convenience stores.

Here it's helpful to ask why customers will buy. Sometimes it's location, sometimes it's simply because they always have. At other times you may be filling an existing need or demand that is so great, sales are almost a given. Sometimes people will buy for convenience, sometimes for price, sometimes because what you offer will help the customer earn more money. Whatever the reason why customers will buy, you should be able to identify it.

When addressing this question, you should give consideration to just how intense the competition is. A West Coast woman intending to enter the fish wholesaling business determined that the market for some of the largest restaurants in the area was very intense, but that small and mid-sized restaurants promised relatively easy entry into the market. In five conversations, she had four tentative commitments from restaurant owners to buy at least some of their seafood from her, if she were to go into business.

When considering whether you can get enough sales,

you should also consider whether special sales, marketing and promotion skills are necessary to be successful in the business. If you don't have them, then logically you'd want to be able to hire someone who did.

And are you selling something people already use, or will you have to convince people to start using your product or service? If you are trying to introduce a new concept, it may take a long time before people accept it to the extent that you can build significant sales. If that is the case, you would have to know how you would be able to support yourself during the "missionary stage," when you are introducing the concept.

Answering this question, of course, is the key to success for most new or small businesses. Statistics over the years continually show that a major cause for the failure of new businesses is a failure to generate sufficient sales. Looking hard and close at this question upfront can sometimes lead you to adopt a different strategy, and become more successful right from the start.

5. Can You Operate at Profit Margins that Will Enable You to Reach Desired Levels of Income?

And How Much Cash Do You Need to Have Upfront, Before the Business Starts to Generate Enough Cash to Support You?

The answer to both of these questions is usually answered by a simple cash flow projection. Envisioning how you will operate, week by week and month by month, you put down figures for the income you expect to receive each month, and the expenses.

A couple on the West Coast proposing to start up a cleaning business did this, and found that their proposed business would indeed be profitable enough to give them the income they wanted, but they would have to plan on losing money the first four months, before starting to make money.

This meant they would need $5000 in cash to tide them over before they could support themselves with earnings from the business. Knowing that ahead of time caused them to wait until they had sufficient funds, and avoid what might have been serious financial problems.

If you don't know how to make a financial projection, don't be concerned. Assistance in this and other areas will be provided. It helps, however, if you can first sit down and figure out how you expect to operate, and the kinds of expenses you expect to incur. Often the best you can do is to make best guess estimates, and in that respect it is often helpful to make two sets of guesses, one conservative and the other optimistic.

When you make an estimate, make a note of the assumption underlying that estimate. In other words, if you estimate printing costs at $200 per month, make a note on what you assumed in order to reach that figure. For example, you may have assumed that you would order the printing of 500 flyers per month, and 300 reprints of an article. By keeping track of your assumptions, if you need to change your figures later, you will know how it will affect operations.

It is important not to overlook expense categories or overestimate profit margins, when putting together financial projections. Here is a helpful list of items to consider.

Sales (Unit Sales)

Lease Income

Bad Checks

Credit Co. Charges

Credit Co. Reversals

Refunds

Commissions

Taxes

Staff Salaries

Casual Labor

Benefits

Outside Contractors

Cost of Goods Sold

Raw Materials

Overhead

Transportation & Storage

Rent and Utilities

Depreciation

Lease Costs

Interest

Travel & Entertainment

Advertising & Promotion

Sales Costs

Printing

Postage

Office Supplies

Insurance

Accounting

License

Memberships

Training

Legal Fees

Bank Charges

6. What Will Your Total Startup Costs Be?

In the previous question we mentioned the cash you would need to support the business before it starts generating sufficient profits to support you. That is only one of the elements in startup capital requirements, however.

In addition, you may have to purchase certain assets, such as equipment, inventory, or a building, and you may have to pay up-front for advertising and marketing materials, licenses, deposits, accounting and legal fees, training, and other items. It is extremely important not to overlook any startup costs, especially if you are cutting it close.

7. Have You Considered the Risks and Tried to Minimize Them?

There is no such thing as a no-risk business, but you can place a business on a continuum from low-risk to high-risk. Giving careful consideration to all the risks up-front can help you to take steps to minimize them. Sometimes it's as simple as buying something like business interruption insurance. But for some risks, the best you can do is make an educated guess.

If you purchase a retail store, for example, you can never be guaranteed that a competitor will not open up down the block in a month or two. You can make your best guess, however, on whether that is likely to happen, based on the size of the existing market, the availability of buildings, the investment required, growth potential for the area, and other factors.

Some of the standard factors to consider when calculating risks, include trends in the area, pending legislation, and any factors that might affect your ability to get a continued supply of materials, or that would affect continued demand for your product or service.

Is the demand for your product or service concentrated in just a few customers? Do you have only one or two sources of supply? Are there any factors that would affect your ability to perform in this business? Is there likely to be greater pressure on your profit margins in the months ahead?

How about the competition? A woman with a tanning salon and exercise tables in the northeast was doing fine for the first year, but three competitors opened up in the second year, forcing her to sell out at a loss. That's direct competition. There is also, "concept competition." A couple that had invested in a small bottled water company met unexpected competition when home water filters became popular in their area.

Are there special skills required to operate your business, and if you don't have them, can you easily hire someone with the right skills? A gas station owner who couldn't replace a skilled mechanic lost a lot of business. Is the proposed business complex, requiring careful management of many different factors? If so, be sure you can manage them.

8. Why Are You Qualified to Run This Business?

Some businesses require a certain type of personality. Is yours suitable? Others require certain experience or abilities if you are truly going to be in control of the business. Do you have that experience or those abilities? Some require an exceptional sales personality.

Others pose a lot of stress. Some require long hours. Others are relatively "lonely" businesses, in that they provide little chance for social interaction. When you consider the nature of your business, and how you would operate day in and day out, it's important to know that this type of business would be compatible with your personality, values, and priorities.

If you're purchasing a business, have you checked with a lawyer and accountant to make certain you and the seller are both getting the best tax advantages? And are you protected in the event sales drop?

It may be preferable to buy assets instead of stock in a company, and if the owner is expected to finance a portion of the purchase price, sometimes the balance due can vary depending upon what happens to sales. Sometimes both the seller and buyer can realize tax advantages if the assets are priced reasonably, and the proper value is assigned to a non-compete agreement, which is often essential for the continued success of a business.

Conclusion

If you're thinking of going into a business, there's probably good reason for it, and a lot of reasons why you are well suited to that particular business. The fastest and most direct way to make it a reality is to get started as soon as possible with an action-oriented plan, which will very quickly bring you up against the reality of that business. You will either become quickly more confident, or realize it wasn't such a good idea.

The first step in putting together that plan is for you to fill out the enclosed worksheet and return it. Don't be concerned about what you don't know. A few conversations and a little firsthand research can often provide all the answers that are needed.

If the success of your business will depend upon selling your talents to prospects, or if you will need to attract investors, then it will also help if you fill out a separate set of forms that provide background information on your experience, strengths, and abilities. The information in those forms may be used to create a brochure about you, a summary of credentials, letters or a resume, as may be required.

(This concludes the reprint of the instructions for the "going into business" forms.)

Daniel T. McAneny

Since 1986, for over a dozen major insurers, Dan has worked one-on-one with over 1900 people on disability. He has helped people at all income levels, in a variety of occupations, in all parts of the U.S.

While Dan started out exclusively in helping people to find new jobs, in recent years the industry has also used him to assist those who want to start or buy a business, or purchase a franchise.

Dan has a broad background in business. It includes manufacturing, banking, advertising, executive job marketing and consulting on corporate growth directions. As a result, he can be effective with almost anyone, from any background. He has scrutinized in depth thousands of careers, gaining insights into many occupations and businesses.

He studied Accounting, Banking and Finance at NYU Graduate School of Business Administration, and his undergraduate degree in Sociology was earned from Holy Cross College in Worcester.

www.ingramcontent.com/pod-product-compliance
Lightning Source LLC
Chambersburg PA
CBHW060858280326
41934CB00007B/1100